FOOD, MEDICINE,
AND THE
QUEST FOR GOOD HEALTH

FOOD, MEDICINE, AND THE QUEST FOR GOOD HEALTH

Nutrition, Medicine, and Culture

NANCY N. CHEN

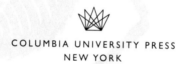

COLUMBIA UNIVERSITY PRESS
NEW YORK

Columbia University Press
Publishers Since 1893
New York   Chichester, West Sussex
Copyright © 2009 Columbia University Press
All rights reserved
Library of Congress Cataloging-in-Publication Data
Chen, Nancy N.
Food, medicine, and the quest for good health:
nutrition, medicine, and culture / Nancy N. Chen.
p. cm.
Includes bibliographical references and index.
ISBN 978-0-231-13484-2 (hard cover : alk. paper) —
ISBN 978-0-231-50891-9 (e-book)
1. Diet therapy—Social aspects.
2. Functional foods—Social aspects.
3. Food habits. 4. Medical anthropology.
I. Title.
RM217.C44   2008
615.8'54—dc22   2008026477

Columbia University Press books are printed on permanent and
durable acid-free paper.
Printed in the United States of America
c 10 9 8 7 6 5 4 3 2

For Sami and Laeti,
who make life immeasurably sweet;
and to Dru,
spice of my life

CONTENTS

CONTENTS

Food and medicine matter immensely to me. I grew up in southern Louisiana, where the local food cultures of Cajun, Creole, African, Spanish, Native American, and southern cooking provided a deeply textured world of foodways, or culinary habits and practices. When they were children my parents did not live in times of plenty; as a result, I have inherited thrifty habits and deeply appreciate sustenance of all sorts. Schools prepared all food from scratch then. My fondest memory of elementary school was arriving to the morning scent of freshly baked bread. At home my parents continued to make the foods of their childhood, so rice was a staple, along with regional Chinese dishes. As immigrants who came to the United States during the golden era of the 1960s, my parents were always curious about American food culture, so we frequently visited cafeterias and po-boy shacks. They rarely denied me or my siblings items that were deemed "bad," such as junk food, fast food, highly sugared cereals, doughnuts, or deep-fried fatty foods. My mother never cooked with written recipes or cookbooks, relying instead on taste. I also learned about food preparation by visiting other friends' homes and by reading the instructions on the box.

How, then, did I come to appreciate food on a continuum with medicine and associate certain foods with nutritional value? It started at home. Instead of relying solely on biomedicine, my mother incorporated her knowledge of Chinese nutritional therapy, which gives food properties according to such factors as the temperature of the food, its dampness, and its bitterness or sweetness. In addition to ready-made ointments and tinctures from her homeland to patch up scrapes, cuts, and infections, my mother brewed ginger in wine or added brown sugar to stewed pears whenever we caught a cold or cough. Stomach troubles meant that our diets would change: we would be put on a strict regimen of rice congee (or porridge), sometimes with a tiny pickled turnip, until our stomachs were better. When stricken with a fever or flu, we were given a changed food regimen as well. My mother would first eliminate spicy or oily foods; then she would slowly reintroduce very plain foods, such as a thin, watery rice porridge. Gradually, as we got better, the gruel became less watery and more like rice. Rice porridge can be a desirable food when we are well. At dim sum restaurants congee is served as a morning meal, and it can be consumed as a late-night snack. For the elderly and young babies with no teeth this can be a nutritious and easily digestible staple. In European desserts rice puddings tend to be sweetened with sugar or honey or made with milk and spices. Decades later, in graduate school, I learned that the recommended WHO (World Health Organization) oral rehydration therapy for diarrhea and starvation was basically watery rice porridge.

As a medical anthropologist, I have come full circle in my study of healing across cultures. I am committed to reimagining and envisioning well-being as part of an integral relationship between eating, thinking, and caring about food and food as medicine. Long before medicines were packaged and sold, people knew about the medicinal value of certain foods. Food is one of the accessible ways in which people experience culture. At the same time, the role of medicine in culture can reveal the values and principles of that culture. In this book I examine the intersections between food and medicine, a relationship that has all too often been obscured because the two are frequently seen as entirely different categories. Thinking about food and medicine as part of a continuum rather than as two separate arenas offers important insights into the consumption of food and the healing process. Moreover, a cultural perspective offers insights into eating and medicating by asking, "What is good food? What is good medicine?" especially in an age of concern about counterfeit medicines, processed foods, and GMOs (genetically modified organisms). Living with industrialized food systems in which the consumer is distanced from the production of food means that we know even less about the healing qualities of food. As notions of nutrition and well-being evolve, framing how different cultures view their food, medicine, and the relationship between the two offers ways through which we can retain that lost knowledge. A cultural perspective can offer ways in which we can appreciate food in all its diversity and make us rethink our medical practices.

Healing foods are intimately linked to culture and its belief systems. In a consumer society most emphasis on food and health care is placed on ensuring a variety of selections. And, to be sure, politics greatly influence the availability of certain foods and medicines. Instead of considering food as medicine as a historical legacy or as a new choice made available through nutraceuticals or genetically engineered drugs, it is important to take into account the intimate connections between healing and culture. Healing foods are deeply embedded in cultural practices, environment, and belief systems. Eating and health care are personal but are also social and political processes. Keeping food and medicine separate has consequences, just as dissolving these boundaries would. Rather than disentangling food and medicine from each other, I try to consider how cultural frameworks may or may not enable a keen understanding of eating and healing as part of a continuum.

Part I examines how contemporary scientific knowledge, social practices, and market interests reframe the medicinal properties of food and how it is consumed. Part II traces the paradox of the increasing distance between food and medicine at the same time that categories of medicine and food intertwine as nutraceuticals or as genetically modified organisms (GMOs) in the contemporary industrial food and pharmaceutical context. Interspersed in the chapters are some recipes that have been served to me for healing purposes. In sum, forms of healing do not necessitate medicating with prescription drugs. Rather, what and how one eats can constitute preventive medicine as well as promote healing.

ACKNOWLEDGMENTS

This book emerged from many lovely meals with family and friends. In southern Louisiana, my parents and brothers instilled in me an appreciation of the pleasures of eating. My mother's stories of healing foods, her medicinal knowledge, and her readings of the *Huangdi Neijing Suwen* (Yellow Emperor's Classic of Internal Medicine) helped pave the way for thinking of food and medicine on a continuum. My godparents in China and their children's generosity made meals restorative and joyful. Innumerable friends, mentors, and families have shared their tables over the years, offering much thought and care. I am especially grateful to Matteo Ames, Kathryn Barnard and Ken Shirriff, Ken K. and Ann Beatty, Yuko and Akira Chiba, Peggy Delaney and Jack Mallory, Melanie Dupuis and Carl Pechmann, Eli Herrera and Dana Hobson, Dana Frank, the Ghasarians, Gary Gray, Scott McMillan, Weiguo Hu, Yueqin Huang, Ann Kingsolver, Robyn Kliger, Paul and Kris Lubeck, Jesus Mejia and Debbie Woods, Laura Nader, M. Todd Ohanian, the Ouyangs, Annapurna and Loki Pandey, C. Alexander Payne, Kelly Pritchett, Gang Qian, Nancy Scheper-Hughes,

Jozseph Schultz and Ann Simonton, Indigo Som and Donna Ozawa, the late Beverly Ramsey, Peter and Judy Thibadeau, Velina Underwood, the Zhangs, and Xinzuo Zhong.

This book was inspired when I lived and worked in Santa Cruz, California, where deep passions for food and medicine are part of daily life. My colleagues Jozseph Schultz, Melanie DuPuis, Melissa Caldwell, Bill Friedlander, Olga Najera-Ramirez, Ravi Rajan, Karen Tei Yamashita, and the AgFood working group have been special companions in food and thought. Students in my classes on Cultures through Food, Medical Anthropology, and Food and Medicine helped frame the chapters. Members of the Asian American Pacific Islander community, especially Nancy Kim, CAAPIS, and APISA, offered moral support and sustenance. Scripps College and Pomona College enabled my family to live under one roof as this manuscript was revised. I am grateful to editor Juree Sondker, who shaped the vision of this book and patiently awaited revisions, despite life events. Jennifer Crewe continued to develop this book with her keen editorial direction. The valuable feedback of three anonymous reviewers made this book much improved. Mary Dearborn's and Cynthia Garver's thoughtful suggestions helped clarify the book's message. I offer heartfelt *rehmet* to Dru C. Gladney, who shared love, laughter, and sustenance though challenging times. Our *ohana* is deeply precious.

This book is dedicated to Sami Chen, whose insight and spirit inspire me to savor life. May she always shine to pave the way for Laetitia Vivian. *Laissez les bons temps rouler!*

Honolulu, Hawaii

FOOD, MEDICINE,
AND THE
QUEST FOR GOOD HEALTH

in his treatise *On Regimen in Acute Diseases*. Similarly, the Chinese Daoist practitioner and pharmacist Sun Simiao (A.D. 581–682) wrote a compendium of herbal medicine, the *Qianjin Yaofang* (*Prescriptions Worth a Thousand Pieces of Gold for Emergencies*) (Li and Li, 2003; Cheng, 2001). Later referred to as the king of medicine, Sun was reputed to have lived 101 years and was widely respected for his compendium. Both practitioners based their findings on empirical observation of herbs or foods that were known to be medicinal. The work of such early physicians offers insights into how medical knowledge can be understood in dietary terms and how dietary practices are integral to medicinal practice. Moreover, the meanings of health and well-being are not just found in formalized medical knowledge; they are also deeply embedded in cultural practices, as well as in attendant social relations.

Cultural Norms of Eating

Food is one of the most universal yet culturally specific material forms. What we eat, how it is prepared and eaten, who is allowed to eat, where we eat, and when we eat are highly enculturated practices. As an anthropologist, I teach my students that one of the most powerful lessons about culture is the way in which cultural beliefs and practices organize everyday life into meaningful categories. These kinds of categories offer important insights about institutions and about the personal meanings that are generated from classification systems in general (Bowker and Starr, 1999).

Anthropology examines both the significance of food in culture and what happens when food is scant or nonexistent and how people respond to such scarcity. During World War II and in the postwar period, Margaret Mead, one of the most well known public anthropologists whose work with children and adolescents transformed conceptions of the life cycle, acted as a national advisor on food and hunger. Her essay on the paradox of hunger in the midst of food surplus, "The Changing Significance of Food," is nearly 40 years old but is still applicable today (Counihan and Van Esterik, 1997). She examines how North American policies shifted from viewing food socially to thinking of it in the context of national security. She argues for a new vision of food in which we address hunger in local contexts in order to make a real contribution to the global struggle for equality. Government and political interventions in the form of food regulations can make a great difference. Since Mead's work in the post–World War II era, Marion Nestle's study of the role of U.S. governmental food policies revealed a shift from an "eat more" to an "eat less" approach (2002). One government intervention during the past decade, for instance, was when the Finnish government encouraged the production and consumption of low-fat dairy products, which led to a significant reduction in national rates of heart disease.[1]

Anthropologists have since focused on different aspects of food, ranging from physical needs to social needs (e.g., those for belonging, etiquette, status, and self-realization). They also study systems of food production and consumption. Sidney Mintz's pathbreaking study of sugar reveals how the desire for sweetness is not always natural but is culturally constructed according to the ways colonialism and class formation produce tastes (1986). In anthropology, two prominent approaches have shaped the study of food and culture. One approach examines how food organizes daily life and resources. For example, studies by physical anthropologists show that primates spend a lot more time looking for better-tasting fruits than simply eating those they can easily gather from the ground (Dominy, 2004). The extra effort says a lot for the value of taste over function: primates do not eat only for survival. In a study of food taboos, Marvin Harris argues that many taboos existed for survival purposes, protecting groups from disease, especially dysentery (1985). Categories of food are based on trial and error, and cultural knowledge based on survival usually consists of practices of hygiene and public health. In an analysis of symbolic categories of purity and pollution, such as the biblical recommendations found in the abominations of Leviticus, where herbivores are considered clean and carnivores unclean, Mary Douglas, a British social anthropologist, does not consider such categorizations as irrational but looks at how qualities attributed to animals reflected human practices of separation and completeness. And rather than considering these approaches oppositional, Douglas argues that both are crucial in thinking about food and even are mutually constitutive: as humans, we eat to live and we live to eat.

Who, What, Where, and When We Eat

Food and medicine have always had a place in the symbolic realm. While contemporary nutritional science emphasizes the material of food, breaking it down into caloric or other energy units, the metaphors of food as fuel can show us how and why some people eat. Thinking about food and medicine in cultural perspective takes into consideration not only how the science of food works but also how notions of food fit into the everyday world. A critical approach to the cultures of food and medicine asks who eats what, where, when, and why. At each of these levels, cultural prescription shapes how certain foods are valued and eaten—or not eaten—at particular times. In earlier centuries, food ideologies grew out of religious prescriptions. Thus, in Catholicism, believers avoid meat on particular days or over certain periods. In many forms of Buddhism, animal flesh is unacceptable as food. Jews and Muslims do not eat pork, and both have restrictions on how foods are prepared.

The forms food and medicines take in a particular culture are greatly influenced by cultural norms. Though nutrition may be available by means of intravenous injection or as dietary supplements, humans prefer foods as they are found in nature or simulate dishes that resemble familiar foods. Astronauts have elaborate freeze-dried meals that are rehydratable to make them look as close as possible to the real thing. By contrast, in futuristic films such as *Brazil* and *The Matrix*, characters eat gray mush for sustenance, suggesting little resemblance to natural foods. Food does more than fuel the body; it also defines us as living cultural beings in the world. So, in a sense, food creates and maintains the boundaries of the social being as well as the individual body. When we consider food, we make choices based on our cultural knowledge and nutritional literacy or awareness of food's innate qualities. Thus, our definitions of food can change when there is cultural contact with other societies.

Culture influences when we eat. We acquire a sense that certain foods and medicines are ingested at certain times. Many societies have a first meal of the day to break the fast from the hours of sleep. In North American households, for instance, families usually don't eat savory leftovers from dinner for breakfast. For some reasons, including a profit motive, Westerners have created a new category, breakfast foods, which includes processed cereals; these were initially created and packaged to make money and promote high-fiber foods over red meat. The creation of foods intended for the start of the day has resulted in the classification of breakfast linked to specific forms of consumption. Yet in places such as Asia, dinner leftovers may be eaten immediately in the morning so that food isn't wasted. If North American diners eat cold pizza and drink soda in the morning, they might well feel an innate sense of transgression. Other ways in which cultural practices determine when we may eat food include religious fasts, which begin and end at specific times. Timing is everything. Many biomedical doctors typically prescribe that certain medicines be "taken with food."

One also has to consider food storage: North American and some European households tend to have larger refrigerators than those in Asia, Latin America, and Africa. Peter Menzel and Faith D'Aluisio's photodocumentary of 30 families around the world and their varied food consumption vividly illustrates differences in the range and amount of foods consumed on a weekly basis (2005). When large amounts of food can be stored for days, and even weeks, families do not need to go shopping as frequently as they must when refrigerators are small or nonexistent. Storage of food and access to it is a crucial part of understanding food consumption.

Culture influences how we eat in different settings. Where we eat or dine changes according to whether we eat at home or in public venues such as cafes, food stalls, or restaurants. Each setting has a different standard for how we eat. Eating in bed, for example, involves rules different from those that might apply to eating in a restaurant, even if the same food is consumed in both places. Contemporary restaurants in Miami and Los Angeles play on notions of transgression and comfort by offering clientele the opportunity to recline on mattresses or oversized pillows while dining. Luis Buñuel's film

The Discreet Charm of the Bourgeoisie (1972) reverses the dining room and the bathroom. An elaborate dining room is filled with guests who converse while sitting on toilet seats around the table. They do everything but eat. Later, when guests wish to eat, they furtively go to the bathroom to consume their food without being seen. This stunning reversal of spaces and the behaviors associated with them shows how we can become accustomed to specific contexts and places in which we eat. Recent venues, such as juice bars that offer shots of wheatgrass or vitamins with fresh-squeezed juice, have transformed how nutrients may be purchased and consumed.

How we eat and the social manners associated with eating indicate a great deal about status, class, gender, religion, culinary ideology, and even nationality. Though many indicators are breaking down because of globalization, cultural factors dictate which foods are consumed with utensils or with hands. Ethiopian restaurants are more common in the United States today, and there it is perfectly acceptable to use fingers rather than any utensils at all. North Americans are sometimes astonished by how Europeans use utensils; all foods, including peas and mashed potatoes, tend to be pushed onto the fork rather than switching knife and fork between left and right hands.

Though hierarchical foodways are significantly less ritualized in modern times, some cultures distinguish who is to eat and in what order. In some Latin American countries, men of the household eat first while women and children eat after them. In other cultures, where old age is revered, such as in Japan, elderly relatives and children are served first and others last. In many religions, devotees do not eat until all forms of prayer and ritual have been conducted. In many regions scarcity may mean that difficult choices must be made about who gets to consume hard-won medicine or food and who does not.

Waiting until everyone is served before beginning to eat is one custom associated with Western dining. At Chinese banquets, one must serve the guest of honor first and then fellow diners before serving oneself. Sociologist Norbert Elias's work on the history of manners offered detailed insight to the eating practices that gave rise to class distinctions in European society (1982). His discussion concurs with Pierre Bourdieu's work (1984), both arguing that cultural prescriptions of how we eat tend to be indicative of our place in the world. Making noise by chewing, swallowing, or burping tends to be taboo at the Western dining table. The Japanese film *Tampopo* (1985) has a revealing scene in which girls in a Japanese finishing school watch a teacher gracefully twirling a forkful of pasta and placing it quietly into her mouth. At the next table they hear a European diner loudly slurping his noodles. When it is their turn to eat, they decide to imitate the Westerner and loudly slurp their pasta as one might a bowl of ramen. The film captures the paradox of clashing cultural practices. Should one slurp one's noodles to express the appreciation of food, or should one slowly twirl the pasta and consume it quietly, as if a member of the upper classes?

Finally, culture influences what we eat. Cultural norms have a great influence on what we consider edible. We may never want to eat snails, worms, bugs, lizards, or other creepy crawly things, for instance; but if they are presented as food options in a society that eats them regularly, we might consider trying such items. Sometimes, in order to avoid offending one's host, the honored guest must eat dishes with exotic and mundane ingredients that transgress cultural and personal boundaries. This practice has become standard fare on certain extreme adventure or reality television shows such as *Fear*

Factor and *Survivor*, in which peer pressure and the desire to win at all costs push contestants to consume animal parts or exotic bugs. The rapid gorging of these items is intended to shock audiences yet at the same time push viewers to reconsider boundaries of what is edible. Entomophagy, the consumption of insects, has recently been touted as an environmentally friendly source of protein ingestion since bugs reproduce more rapidly than domesticated animals. In some cuisines, larvae are integrated into dishes such as silkworm broth in southern China or casu marzu, a Sardinian cheese that has been fermented with larvae. While the intentional consumption of larvae, grubs, and other forms of insects tends to be considered an exotic practice, the more mundane everyday consumption of insect parts in cereals, fruits, peanut butter, and spices is often overlooked.

A cross-cultural taboo found in most of today's societies is cannibalism. Many of the taboos surrounding cannibalism exist for social purposes, primarily to make us distinguish human from animal. Eating human flesh is highly transgressive, but historical examples show that sometimes eating human flesh has been considered necessary for survival or for ritual purposes. For the ancient Aztecs, consuming the flesh of the enemy in human sacrifice was a ritual of power. It was also a way to provide protein for a growing population and armed forces when food sources were insufficient. Also, as Shirley Lindenbaum discovered, in areas of Papua New Guinea, tribal members once considered it to be fulfillment of an important funeral ceremony to have one's relatives eat one's flesh (1979). In cases in which survival was at issue, such as the ill-fated group at Donner Pass in Nevada and that of an airplane crash in the Andes, eating dead human flesh was necessary to survive and thus deemed a gruesome exception.

Sensory Perceptions and Eating

The senses greatly influence how we experience food and medicine. Industrialized food and medical systems can obscure the origins of these categories. Sensory knowledge about one's food or medicine was an important part of the therapeutic process in the three ancient world systems of medicine: Greco-Islamic, Ayurvedic, and Chinese. In each system, food and medicinal items had certain energetic qualities. Recognizing the innate quality of foods and matching these to the needs of the patient whose body was out of balance were integral to all three systems.

Smell is perhaps the sense that is most linked to memory and place. Smell is not just a sense that determines taste; it is also a powerful force that stimulates desire and may even overwhelm the other senses. In the past decade, aromatherapy has emerged as an alternative healing practice, as well as a new product to be touted to consumers. Some stores disperse scents of freshly baked bread or apple pie to encourage shoppers to linger and buy more. Smells are also important for distinguishing between edible and inedible foods. Herbal medicine stores frequently have a wide variety of pungent odors. The preparation of herbal medicines may include cooking plants into liquid form or distilling essences with alcohol, which often creates an odor. Yet biomedical pills and tablets are prepared in ways that deemphasize smells considered to be more palatable. The absence of smells further distances medicine from food.

The visual presentation of food is perhaps the most emphasized. Vision tends to be privileged over our other faculties. Some cultures have elaborate dishes that look like something else, like sugar skulls or chocolate rabbits. In Japan, people are exposed to plastic versions of food (which are even more expensive than the real thing); there are also Thai fruit and vegetable carvings, European marzipan, and Buddhist vegetarian foods that are made to taste and look like meat. The practice of adding salt, vitamins, coloring, or preservatives to chocolates, drinks, and other foods has long helped to disguise less-appealing textures, colors, and smells.

Culture may shape not only how a food looks but also how it feels. Limpness or firmness and oiliness or dryness greatly determine how appetizing the dish is. In North American society, for instance, if a diner ordered a steak medium rare and it turned out to be well done, he or she might consider the dish ruined. The cultural preferences of the producer of food and the consumer's need are directly related. The smoothness of tablets or pills is a factor contributing to their uniformity. Finally, taste may determine whether we reject a food item. Taste is highly individual while it is also culturally prescribed. The kinds of tastes can be divided according to such qualities as bitterness, sweetness, sourness, or saltiness, and different cuisines may emphasize or combine distinctive tastes. When at a dinner with Chinese friends, a good part of the time is spent in recognizing different flavors and remarking on them. How did the cook, for instance, make eggs cooked in vinegar taste like fresh crab? Cultural notions of taste influence whether bitterness should be masked. Biomedical pills and syrups have long included sugar or other additives to mask the taste of the medicine. By contrast, herbal medicines tend to have strong flavors and aftertastes that are not hidden with bubblegum flavors.

Overview of the Book

Food and medicine have been intertwined for many centuries, along both the Spice Routes and the Silk Road. Healing foods are recognized in the three major medicinal traditions: Chinese, Ayurvedic, and Greco-Islamic. These medical systems rely on food to purify, tone, and heal the body, and they prevail on dietary prescriptions to do so. These three systems, which have survived for centuries, inform nutritional contemporary beliefs and practices. Certain commodities, such as spices, sugar, and salt, were invaluable not only as seasonings or preservatives but also as medicinal entities in their own right. Finally, certain foods were considered to be good for having a long life. In these systems, analyzing the humoral principles of food (and of bodies) could contribute to longevity. Place, time, and production, for instance, determine what we call comfort food.

Contemporary scientific knowledge, social practices, and market interests determine the medicinal properties of foods and their consumption. Nutraceuticals and genetically modified organisms (GMOs) represent the transformation of the consumption of medicine by way of blurring the boundaries between medicine and food. The current market in medicines consumed as food is a booming industry. (Consider, for example, Viactiv calcium in chocolate form and the vitamins contained in Odwalla drinks.) The promises of nutraceuticals inform the impact that the pharmaceutical industry has on daily life. Our society has tipped the balance in favor of genetically modified (GM) foods and genetically engineered (GE) drugs. Though genetically modified foods are actively resisted in Europe, over one-half of the processed foods in the United States include GM ingredients. Moreover, in India and China, GM crops have been developed with the Malthusian premise that GMOs will prevent widespread hunger and dependency. Farmers in these countries are told that these crops require fewer pesticides. But do GMO crops decrease the need for pesticides? Current cultural discourses involve GMOs, notions of purity, and the transformation of food into medicine.

Nutritional literacy and awareness of the intimate linkages between food and medicine are critical for primary care. Eating for health involves thinking and reimagining the historical and social linkages between food and medicine. A cultural approach entails paying close attention not only to the contexts of production but also to how foodways and nutritional knowledge shape the contours of medicine. In addressing these links, it is my hope that the sensual pleasures of eating and healing can be understood as forms of cultural knowledge and practices that can be lost, recovered, or transformed.

PART ONE

Food as Medicine

CHAPTER ONE

Healing Foods and Longevity

Traditional medical systems offer extensive documentation of the connection between food and medicine. Ancient Chinese, ancient Greek, Islamic, and Ayurvedic medicines have shared systemic views of the body, its properties or humors, and notions of energy and nutrition. The preservation of health and extension of life, particularly for elites, was a common goal of many practitioners for their clientele in these early societies. Healing foods, or foods that can be eaten raw or cooked in combination with other items, were a critical component of maintaining well-being. In this sense, the "doctoring" of foods—whether with spices or herbs—was a basic form of preventive medicine that all traditional systems of healing have shared. The preparation of medicinal dishes may involve a process of cooking or distilling to tap the healing properties of the herbs or spices.

Spices occupied part of a broader spectrum of beliefs about foods that were considered to have specific medicinal properties. Food and medicine were rarely separated into different categories; instead, the continuum of beliefs considering food as medicine and medicine as food spanned the globe. The early trade in spices along various routes of the Silk Road contributed greatly to their use in both food and medicine in all of the major medical traditions. Spicing up foods not only introduced new flavors but also made the use and consumption of spices an integral part of medicinal dishes that have come to be part of foodways. The consumption of food and spices to purify, tone, and heal the body or extend life have been addressed in ancient Chinese, Greco-Islamic, and Ayurvedic medicine. These traditional medical systems continue to be practiced and inform contemporary beliefs about diet and nutrition. The history of medicine offers a way to see in a vivid and enlightening way the healing properties of food within a larger context. Scholars have indicated that practitioners, rather than thinking of these medical systems as distinct or separate, were engaged with various translations of sources in an ongoing exchange of knowledge.

The scholarship on traditional medicine has primarily compared ancient Chinese and Greek medicine (Kuriyama, 1999; Lloyd, 1996; Lloyd and Sivin, 2002). Few discussions have comparatively analyzed the diet therapies of these systems. These forms of traditional medicine share several distinguishing elements: secularization of medical knowledge from spiritual forms of healing, emphasis on regulation of hygiene and nutrition, and notions of balance with the environment. Secularized medicine offered the means to distinguish theories of healing with food, climate, region, and taste from folk or heterodox spiritual practices. Systematic correlations of food, medicine, and their effects were key to classifying medicine as part of institutional practice rather than remaining in the realm of charismatic healers. Diseases, ailments, and plagues were considered to be deeply enmeshed with a person's social and political milieu. Body and self were intimately tied to environmental elements such as air, water, heat, cold, and dampness. Through classification systems of the four humors, or fluids that influence the body's health, certain body types were correlated to how foods were processed. Properties of food such as taste or texture and their effects varied differently, depending on digestion of the food and its incorporation into the body. Principles of humoral theory, based on the correlation of flavors with body types, were common to all three systems. Examining the links between food and medicine in ancient Chinese, Greco-Islamic, and Ayurvedic medicine leads us to rethink present-day diet-related concerns such as cardiovascular disease, diabetes, and obesity.

Chinese Food and Medicine

Food therapy, known as *shi liao* in Mandarin, has a long history in Chinese medicine. Eating each meal or specific food items with an intent to maintain health, promote vitality, or alleviate illness is the central principle of food therapy and can be an integral part of daily life, according to this system. The practice is based on an extensive classification of foods in specific food groups, tastes, and characteristics. Based on these categories, food therapy also entails the preparation of foods with healing herbs or spices that then become medicinal dishes. Such practice offers a way to conceptualize food and medicine on a continuum rather than as separate entities. This knowledge permeates contemporary Cantonese foodways, which many scholars, medical practitioners, and consumers note for adherence to the balance of flavors, tastes, and medicinal healing principles that extend back to the *Huangdi Neijing* (Yellow Emperor's Classic

of Internal Medicine). The consumption of rice congee or porridge (*jook* in Cantonese) is a prime example of traditional Chinese food therapy that has persisted in modern-day Cantonese tradition.

The emphasis on food therapy offers an important way
to look at Chinese medicine itself. Rather than thinking of
the contemporary system of healing as the direct descen-
dant of a unified system, it is useful to think of Chinese medicine as having many diverse roots and extensions. Contemporary Chinese medicine incorporates a range of diagnostic and
therapeutic approaches, including pulse and tongue diagnosis, acupuncture, herbal medicine, moxibustion (or burning a
substance on the skin), massage, and Qigong (or Chi Kung; a
practice of postures and breathing to cultivate energy). Medical theories about the body abound, including classifications
according to yin and yang, the five elements, the zang fu organs, and the meridian channels. Diet unifies all of these theories by incorporating many of their conceptions of the body
in the healing process. Within traditional Chinese medicine,
diet therapy was considered to be the first line and the high-
est form of medicine.

FOUNDATIONS OF CHINESE DIET THERAPY

The legend of Shen Nong, or the "divine farmer," is one story
of the beginning of diet therapy. A deity and one of the three
mythical rulers in Chinese tradition, Shen Nong is considered
to be the founder of agriculture and herbal medicine. He ob-
served the effect of various plants that animals consumed. According to folklore, he discovered the potential qualities associated with plants and herbs by tasting each one. Once, when

---

RICE PORRIDGE

Ingredients: rice and water

You may make this porridge with already cooked rice and water or start from scratch. Short-grain white rice yields thicker gruel than long-grain white rice; brown rice is generally not used for porridge. The thicker gruel is more palatable, but the elderly and young children are frequently served a thinner gruel.

Rice porridge may be served plain or with pickled vegetables. Some porridges have specific ingredients designed for particular conditions. For postpartum women, for example, the porridge may be prepared in a chicken or fish broth with garnishes of ginger and green onions.

---

poisoned by an herb, the divine farmer foraged about until he found another herb that remedied it. The *Shen Nong Ben Cao Jing* of the Han dynasty (206 B.C.–220 A.D.) documents the properties of several hundred plants (Yang, 1998). The legend and the documents attributed to the divine farmer indicate how the earliest forms of medicine were inseparable from plants eaten as food.

Another foundation of early Chinese medicine is based on Daoist philosophy and ritual practice. This strand of practice has been referred to as an unofficial form of folk medicine and was characterized as superstitious in state documents that favored a consolidated form of Chinese medicine. Recent scholarship on local and popular practices, however, reveal how prominent Daoist practices were in daily life and medicine (Dean, 1993). Daoist beliefs about the body included a range of dietary practices that enhanced the way of the Dao and its energy known as qi (chi). The body was thought to live in relation to its environment, such that qi flowed in humans, plants, animals, and physical spaces. Specific foods became intimately linked to different rituals and holidays based on categories of associated qi energy. Moreover, Daoists believed that internal alchemy could prepare a body for immortality. Cinnabar was considered to be an exalted substance, its transformation in the body conferring immortality. By contrast, grains and cereals were considered to pollute the body as a spiritual vessel, so abstinence from these items and fasting in general were important steps toward extending life in Daoist thought.

The nutritionist or diet therapist was considered to be the highest-ranking person in the Chou dynasty (1028–480 B.C.) emperor's court (Anderson, 1988: 229). During this period, foods were grouped according to five flavors (pungent, sweet, sour, bitter, and salty) and five smells (fragrant, rancid, scorched, rotten, and putrid) associated with the five elements: earth, metal, fire, wood, and water. There were also five foods—grains, fruits, animals, vegetables, and organs—where the flavors were imparted. The medical classic *Huangdi Neijing Suwen* says:

> Where the five flavors enter:
> Sour enters the liver.
> Acrid enters the lung.
> Bitter enters the heart.
> Salty enters the kidneys.
> Sweet enters the spleen. (Unschuld, 2003: 301)

Humoral medical theory was an important part of Chinese medicine. The humors were based on a system of four properties associated with foods: hot, cold, wet, and dry. Different food items have varying degrees of heat, coolness, dampness, or dryness. These were not always literal qualities but were based on the perceived effects of a substance on the body. The qualities of food could also be characterized in terms of yin and yang principles. Yin was considered to have cooling effects, in which the body's energy level or metabolism was lowered. Cooling foods, including barley, cucumber, mung beans, green vegetables, watermelon, most fruits, crab, and green tea, were thought to tend to have higher water content and thus encourage the restoration of water in the body. Yang foods, by contrast, heated up or increased body metabolism. Heating foods included ginger, garlic, pepper, onions, scallions, alcohol, coffee, black tea, trout, chicken, lamb, dog, pineapple, longan (dragon's eye lychee), dates, plums, pomegranates, peaches, and cherries. Such foods were thought to have a higher fat or protein content, enabling the body to be more energetic. Neutral foods included rice, wheat, corn, soy, red beans, carrots, yams, potatoes, olives, lotus seeds, beef, goose, quail, eel, turtle, jellyfish, abalone, and jasmine tea. Several items, such as pineapple, corn, and abalone, are New World products, but Chinese medicine now includes these new foods.

Combinations of foods with different properties could promote or restore balance in a person's health. Often the principle of oppositions demonstrated that heat could counteract conditions induced by cooling or dampness. Most therapeutic foods, however, were based on a congruence between appearance, texture, and effect. Remedies for circulatory and nervous disorders called for the use of sinuous, slithery animals such as snake or fish to enhance agility of movement. Diet therapy continues to be a significant part of Chinese medicine, often referred to as traditional Chinese medicine (TCM) in the United States.[1] Systematic correspondence of

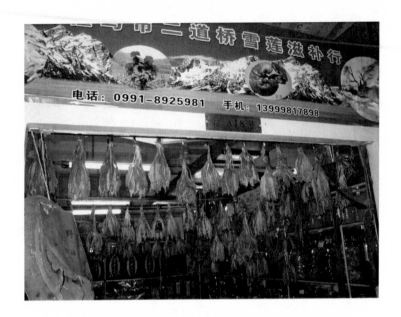

Uighur medicine stall, Urumqi, Xinjiang, 2004

foods with humors or organs is tied to overall body practices that were believed to extend health and life. Foods could restore qi, enhance blood flow, balance yin and yang, and prevent diseases.

USE OF HERBS

The use of herbs in Chinese cooking was intended primarily to promote balance or to transform ingredients into a medicinal dish. The enhancement of flavor was a secondary effect of such preparations. Herbs were frequently combined with foods for strengthening the body. Like foods, herbs also had yin (cooling) or yang (heating) properties. Cassia (Chinese cinnamon) was cooling, ginseng was heating, and licorice was neutral. Though cassia was a cooling substance, it was a tonic used to treat nausea, flatulence, and diarrhea. Chinese cassia is often used in combination with other spices to become what is referred to as five-spice powder, mostly used for stewing fruits and meats.

Ginseng (*Panax*) was noted in a variety of medical texts for its promotion of energy and health. The root of this herb is reputed to have many properties related to longevity, as well to sexual appetite. The root is noted in Chinese medicine for its ability to vitalize the five organs, soothe nerves, and promote overall well-being. Medicinal dishes that include ginseng can be found in Chinese and Korean foodways. Chinese medicinal food recipes may include ginseng in combination with chicken broth as a restorative dish. It is also common to find ginseng steeped in wine, which is consumed for its warming and therapeutic qualities. Though more commonly associated as a flavoring for candies, licorice root has long been valued for its soothing properties. It provides relief for inflammation by enhancing the mucosal lining of the stomach. In combination with honey, it is a principle ingredient of Chinese cough syrups. Because of its neutral quality as a tonic, licorice is used to balance other herbs and spices.

USE OF ANIMAL PARTS

Often in combination with herbs, animal parts were also considered medicinal and were used in food therapy. The more mythical, rare, or strong the animal was considered to be, the more likely it would affect longevity and virility. People in many cultures believe in the powers of animals and may include animal parts in healing rituals, or they may consume specific animals for particular events or holidays. The incorporation of animal parts into medicinal dishes as food therapy is extensively noted in Chinese medicine. Deer antlers, bear paws, and snake bile, among other animal products, are used in both Chinese herbal medicine and in medicinal recipes. Belief in the healing and often aphrodisiac qualities of medicinal foods continues well into the present. After economic reforms in mainland China that gave citizens more money, people visited wild game restaurants that offered menus with exotic animal ingredients.

Such restaurants, particularly in southern China, became subject to the scrutiny of state officials during the SARS (severe acute respiratory syndrome) epidemic in 2004. A number of such restaurants were closed when several workers were diagnosed with SARS. Particular species, such as the civet cat, a kind of mongoose, were cited as carriers of the SARS virus and were therefore culled, in addition to being banned in markets. This animal is often harvested for its musk secretions and is consumed in winter as a delicacy for its heating properties.

The killing of wild animals to meet increased demand for exotic ingredients has been a concern for many animal rights activists over the past decade. Bears, mostly endangered in Asia, are sought for the medicinal effects of the bile from their gall bladders. This substance is used in Chinese medicine as a remedy for fever, convulsions, and hemorrhoids. The trade in bear bile and other parts has led many animal rights groups to question cultural and medicinal practices that lead to the consumption of these animals. Depending on the country, sanctions against the trade in wild game and endangered species are imposed.

Ancient Greek, Galenic Humoral, and
Islamic Food and Medicine

HIPPOCRATES

Greek and Islamic medicine were both influential for medieval European medicine. Ancient Greek medicine is attributed to Hippocrates, who practiced during the fifth century B.C. Hippocrates' views on medicine were distinct from of those ritual specialists, who considered illness to be caused by supernatural rather than natural influences. Building on an extensive base of scientific observation from Aristotle and other scholars in Greece from the sixth century B.C., Hippocrates wrote extensively on natural phenomena to address the connection between environment, disease, and health. His treatise "On Airs, Waters, and Places" offered an early examination of the critical relationship between human bodies and pathogens. The legacy of Hippocratic medicine was extensive, influencing not only Roman medicine but also Islamic and even Ayurvedic and Unani medical theory. The Hippocratic Corpus was a collection of treatises linked to the philosopher/healer; more likely, they originated in various medical practitioners on the island of Cos in the eastern Aegean.

Though mostly known for the Hippocratic oath, still invoked in many American medical schools, Hippocratic writings covered a broad range of subjects pertaining to medicine, including fractures, head injuries, hemorrhoids, ulcers, and epidemics, as well as acute disease, ecology, prognosis, and surgery. The core of this system focused on diet and the natural causes of disease (Lloyd, 2003). The elements of earth, air, fire, and water correlated with the four humors of phlegm, blood, yellow bile, and black bile. The Hippocratic aphorisms offer insight to the prevalent beliefs about the properties of food during the classical Greek period. Observations on the relationship between food and disease were frequently noted; dietary restriction was promoted as the key to health. In the early twenty-first century, raw food enthusiasts and natural healing promoters claim the Hippocratic diet as an inspiration for cleansing and invigorating the body.

GALEN

Hippocratic medicine continued to be practiced for centuries, influencing generations of healers. Perhaps the most famous interpreter of the Hippocratic approach was Galen (129–200 A.D.), a physician in the Roman Empire. Galenic medicine in Rome during the second and third centuries A.D. extended humoral theory in more detail. In his essays "On the Powers of Foods," Galen used classical medical ideas about food and diet to address how nutrition was central to medicinal practice. Book I addressed the properties of cereals, Book II considered those of various fruits and vegetables, and Book III distinguished those of different animals. Such knowledge was on the frontlines of medicine at that time (Galen, 2000). Citing Hippocrates on the necessity of observation, Galen noted how different foods pass through the body at different rates. Drugs were to be used as a second resort, and surgery would only be considered as a last resort.

IBN SINĀ

Medical knowledge from the Hippocratic Corpus traveled widely and was translated into several different languages.

Scholar/practitioners of early Islamic medicine wrote extensive commentaries on the Hippocratic oath and other ancient Greek treatises. From the third to the ninth centuries, most of the key Greek and Roman medical writings had been translated into Arabic, while additional translations appeared in Persian, Sanskrit, and Syriac. These works preserved the classic theories of food, medicine, and the body, which would eventually be translated into Latin. Moreover, during the medieval period, the infusion of new views of diseases and their cures enabled a proliferation of scientific medical practices based on observation and experimentation. Such a foundation became the basis for the earliest medical colleges and hospitals across the Islamic caliphate, particularly in Cairo, Damascus, and Baghdad. Anatomy, physiology, and the study of drugs were among the many contributions of traditional Islamic medicine.

Ibn Sinā (or Avicenna) has been referred to as the doctor of doctors. In the tenth century A.D., Ibn Sinā compiled existing medical knowledge from Greek into Arabic and added his own findings from clinical practice, observation, and experimentation. Ibn Sinā's work, *al-Qanun al-Tibb*, or the Canon of Medicine, synthesized Greek and Arabic views on illness, hygiene, anatomy, and drugs (1996). This encyclopedic text comprised five books and eventually became translated into Latin, which was foundational for later medical works in European medicine. The consideration of health always included the importance of food as the primary form of medicine, diet being a critical path to health and holiness. The link between health and the state was most visible in the clientele of famous physicians such as Ibn Sinā, Hippocrates, and Chinese court physicians. State patronage has always been critical to the practice of traditional medicine. Ibn Sinā's treatment of several rulers and attention to their continued health made it possible for him to pursue his medical career despite unstable times.

PROPHETIC TRADITIONS

Another strand of Islamic medicine that continues today is prophetic medicine, based on Quranic interpretations for physical and spiritual guidance in health matters. While eschewing Galenic and Hippocratic sources in prophetic medicine, many notions of heat, cold, and moisture in relation to food significantly overlapped with these foundations of Islamic medicine. Various scholars and texts incorporated Quranic references with prophetic traditions to address a broad range of diagnoses according to divine law. Diet was considered to be a critical element of spiritual well-being.

Various prophetic guides on medical treatment refer to the stomach as the center of disease. Simple foods were thought to have healthy uses. Dates, for instance, were considered to be "food, medicine, and a fruit," useful especially for those dwelling in hot climates (Ibn Qayyim, 1994: 65–66). Cucumbers as a cooling food also provided important balance in one's diet. Abstinence was another key healing element. In the early stages of illness, abstinence from certain foods was considered to be key in preventing relapse or further degeneration. Boiled barley, in water and porridge, was also considered to be a nutritious source, as in Galen's treatise on barley soup. Barley water, in particular, was considered to be medicinal in both Persian and Indian texts. According to Francoise Aubaile-Sallenave's linguistic and cultural/geographical analysis of barley, "Kishk, or kishka, or kishbab, is the barley preparation of which all medieval scholars speak. They were clearly under the influence of

Greek medicine which considered *ptisana*, 'barley water,' as a true panacea" (2000: 14). Rather than looking to foods merely for their powerful effects, prophetic medicine also addressed the moral and ethical dimensions of food in its preparation, consumption, and digestion. In this way foods maintained both the body and soul.

UNANI MEDICINE

Unani medicine (*tibb*) is a legacy of Hippocratic and Islamic medicine that continues to be practiced extensively in India and Pakistan. Using the theories and texts of medical practitioners Galen, al-Razi (Rhazes), Ibn Sinā (Avicenna), and Ibn Nafis, Unani complemented traditional medicine in Egypt, Syria, Iraq, Persia, India, and China. During the thirteenth to nineteenth centuries A.D., Unani practitioners flourished under the protection of the sultanate as state scholars and court physicians. During this period, experimentation with local Indian herbs and drugs became part of the medical system.

Unani uses the theory of the four humors: blood (hot and moist), phlegm (cold and moist), yellow bile (hot and dry), and black bile (cold and dry), which correspond to the four temperaments—sanguine, phlegmatic, choleric, and melancholic (Azmi, 1995). Depending on a person's constitution, humoral balance was determined by proper diet and digestion. Preventing illness entailed careful attention to the equilibrium of various environmental and physical states. Unani diagnosis also included pulse reading, as well as examination of urine and stool specimens. Various therapies include physical regimens (such as massage, cupping, purging, and exercises); diet therapy that regulates the amount and type of foods eaten; and drug therapy, mostly using herbs and plant compounds. Tonics—restorative or invigorating agents, usually in liquid form—are very common in this system. Though Unani medicine classifies herbs as hot and dry (somewhat unlike their role in Chinese medical classification), many herbal tonic drinks are marketed today as a source of refreshment and cooling (Bright, 1998).

Ayurveda and Healing Foods

Renewed interest over the past decade in Indian cultural practices such as yoga has also turned the focus on Ayurveda as an alternative traditional medical system to biomedicine (Alter, 2005). Ayurveda can be translated as the knowledge (*veda*) of life (*ayur*) and longevity. A South Asian medical system that is also based on humoral theory, Ayurveda resembles its Chinese and Greek counterparts. While Greek and Roman classifications of foods were based on empirical observation of their effects, Ayurvedic approaches offered more dietary and therapeutic categories, which considered the energetic qualities of body and environment (Nair and Monohan, 1998). What a person consumed, whether plant or animal, had specific qualities, such as aroma, essence, and energies, that were imparted to the consumer and influenced his or her humoral interactions. The three major Ayurvedic texts that continue to influence contemporary practice include the *Caraka-samhita*, *Susruta-samhita*, and *Astanga-hrdaya-samhita*.

Ayurveda evolved from Hindu spiritual beliefs and philosophy, with much influence from Buddhist monastic traditions. As in Chinese medical cosmology, the personal being was a microcosm of the broader universe, which had both ecological and ethical dimensions. Focusing on wholesome daily activities, including diet, hygiene, and other routines, would lead to an ideal, holy, and healthy life. Health was thought to come from a dynamic balance; ongoing adjustments of the humors—air, bile, phlegm, and blood—could enable self-knowledge and constitutional well-being. Contemporary Ayurveda practitioners consider a person's body type, seeking to balance the dynamic forces (*doshas*) of *veta*, *pitta*, and *kapha* (Fields, 2001: 80).

Cooking and combining foods were of particular import in Ayurvedic healing. Through combinations of foods, one could achieve the perfection (*samskara*) of remedies and prescriptive enhancement. Meats on their own, for instance, do not have the flavor, intensity, or therapeutic qualities that they do when combined with particular herbs, spices, or other food items. Combinations achieved through cooking offer ways to create more concentrated essences of foods with particular qualities. Whereas the Hippocratic Corpus was concerned with classifying various animals and natural history, Ayurvedic traditions developed a more elaborate focus on the interplay between various humors and the qualities of different foods. Eating foods incongruent with one's bodily makeup could do great harm. Francis Zimmerman's study (1987) on the classification of animals and natural history indicates that the Indian Ayurvedic emphasis on humors and savors is deeply rooted in cultural knowledge of ecology.

What Happened to the Humors?

In this overview of early medicine and the critical role of diet in therapy, it is clear that most traditional systems of medicine had similar views on the human constitution and the need for balance between bodies and environment. These systems viewed food, first, as preventive medicine, and second, as a treatment for ailments. They categorized foods according to their humoral properties and analyzed them according to their influences on digestion. Properties of heat, cold, moisture, and dryness mattered more than taste or texture.

Given the centrality of diet and nutrition to traditional notions of health, the erasure of humoral theory and the shift from nutritional therapy to allopathic forms of treatment in contemporary biomedicine is instructive. During the eighteenth and nineteenth centuries, medicine in the West increasingly emphasized scientific investigation by way of gross anatomy, as dissections became allowed and then accepted as a norm. An emphasis on pathology and specialization in specific systems of the body also transformed views of the body. It would be easy to lament the disappearance of humoral theory. Instead, the persistence of traditional medicines in many parts of the world, in spite of biomedical practice, indicates how food and beliefs about the constitution of bodies remain central to medical practice.

Consideration of how traditional medical systems deem food to be a central component of both harmful pathology and potential relief—even life extension—offers insight into contemporary medicine and how responses to long-term health needs can be approached. The leading causes of disease and mortality in Western countries, as well as in developing nations—cancer, heart disease, and stroke—are greatly influenced by diet. In 2003, the U.S. Centers for Disease Control and Prevention revised its view on obesity, which is practically epidemic in the American populace. In Western medical schools, nutrition is barely represented in the curriculum. Poor diet and lack of access to nutritious foods can be the primary or often secondary contributors to many pathological conditions. Rather than simply adopting a Hippocratic diet, consuming Chinese medicinal dishes, or imbibing an Ayurvedic or Unani tonic in response to pathology, it is important to consider food and medicine in a wider cultural context. In many instances, a quick cure for illness and disease may not always be possible. Instead, a more thorough appreciation of the environmental and social conditions that influence knowledge of and access to food as medicine over an extended period is fundamental to well-being. Eating well from a humoral perspective may entail eating with the properties of foods based on environment and seasons in mind.

Spicing Up Foods as Medicine

When I was growing up in my mother's house, there were spices you grated and spices you pounded, and whenever you pounded spice and garlic or other herbs, you used a mortar. Every West Indian woman worth her salt had her own mortar.

Audre Lorde, *Zami: A New Spelling of My Name*, 1982

Step into any kitchen, or any place where food is prepared, and you will usually find a spot where spices and dried herbs are stored. (Herbs are considered a subset of spices.) Depending on the ethnic foods prepared in the household, additional spices, salt, and sugar might be stored in jars near the stove. The ubiquitous spice cabinet can even come prepackaged with uniform containers filled with cinnamon, pepper, cardamom, rosemary, thyme, coriander, and cumin readily available at stores or through mail-order catalogs. Such an assemblage may seem ordinary and even taken for granted as part of daily life. Yet, as historians and other scholars of food have discovered, spice racks are anything but ordinary. Key transformations in trade and consequently in taste made such materials available and desirable. Merchants and traders in spices made vast fortunes, anticipating, it could be argued, the contemporary oil trade. Spices, often offered as tribute or gifts, were perhaps the earliest form of medicine. Categorized as food-related seasonings today, spices, sugar, and salt were once, in different times and places, considered essential for medicinal purposes, becoming highly prized commodities.

Spices, salt, and sugar are intimately intertwined with the stories of ancient trade routes, newfound tastes, and the rise of industrial food systems. These items were used as currency, becoming synonymous with words representing worth and value. The history of these material entities and their circulation has been a focus of many book-length studies of particular foods, including Mark Kurlansky's *Salt* (2002b). At different times, these ingredients were regarded as healthy—and essential to a good diet—or, alternatively, unhealthy.

Spices were accepted as a form of currency to pay rent or taxes in many trading cities. In this early period of globalization, traders sought different routes to avoid what was initially the Arab monopoly on spices. The history of the spice trade reflects the exclusive access to specific routes and thus to markets for certain spices that various nations have secured in turn. First Arabs dominated the spice trade, and then, in succession, Turks, Italians, Spaniards, the Portuguese, the Dutch, and the French. Finally, English merchants came to dominate the trade.

The Middle East saw the earliest documentation of spices, used in embalming, perfumes, incenses, and medicines. Arabian traders quickly established a monopoly on spices that would last two millennia. Spices were also integral to notions of the good life in Roman times when people began to consume

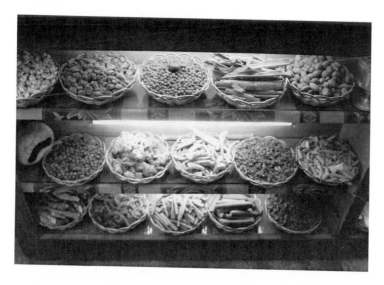

Assorted spices in Egyptian spice market, Istanbul, 2006

them, adding them as luxurious elements to food, wine, medicine, and even cosmetics. J. Innes Miller's 1969 study of the spice trade from 29 B.C. to A.D. 641 traces how the saying "all roads lead to Rome" was literally true for spices. Various trade routes across deserts, mountains, or seas brought spices from Asia to the Roman Empire. Romans used spices as aromatic substances, often added in copious amounts. Spiced wines and foods were provided for guests in sumptuous displays of wealth and excess. The emergence of taste as an indicator of status (because access to these items was available mainly to the rich) fueled the spice trade.

The availability of spices in various forms (leaves, flowers, seeds, roots, branches, twigs, or bark) depended on the politics of the spice trade and people's knowledge of the uses of various substances. Traders carried spices over long distances together with other items, such as silk, gems, and precious metals. The abundant products of the Spice Islands (the Moluccas in Indonesia) were conveyed to Europe by way of China and India. The overland trade routes included the famed Silk Road from China, with a branch to the north and one to the south. The overseas Spice Route included ports and warehouses in China, India, Ceylon (Sri Lanka), Indonesia, the Molucca Straits, southern Arabia, Egypt, and East Africa. Either by land or by sea, all routes held potential dangers, whether natural or human. Though distances by land were shorter, overseas routes were preferable due to the greater number of ports and the more lucrative gains made with each stop.

CASSIA AND CINNAMON

Cassia, or Chinese cinnamon, is perhaps the oldest spice, mentioned in a number of ancient texts in Chinese and Greek. Though the words "cassia" and "cinnamon" are frequently used interchangeably, the two are different varieties of the *Cinnamomum* tree: *C. aromaticum* and *C. zeylanicum*. Cassia bark is darker and coarser, while cinnamon bark is subtler and more often used in sweet dishes. Cassia was used in China for medicinal purposes, as well as in cooking. Many Daoist texts refer to cassia or cinnabar as the elixir of life. A primary ingredient of five-spice powder, cassia was also used by the Egyptians in embalming because of its antiseptic and preservative qualities. Because the fragrant bark traveled the longest distance of any spice, it was also the most valuable cargo. On the "cinnamon route" between Indonesia and Madagascar, traders studied monsoon patterns to traverse the waters with their precious goods.

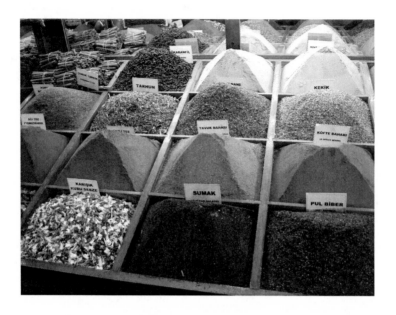

Bins of cinnamon stick, curry powder, and red pepper in
Egyptian spice market, Istanbul, 2006

Cinnamon is believed to have antiseptic qualities and is considered useful for indigestion, diarrhea, and menstrual cramps. Its oil is used as a mosquito repellent. Recent research indicates cinnamon may help with type 2 diabetes because of its insulin-like properties. A *Health Day* news release on April 22, 2004, reported on lab findings from University of California at Santa Barbara researcher Don Graves on the effect of cinnamon on diabetic mice.

PEPPER

Pepper is another aromatic substance that traveled long distances from Asia. Though cinnamon was held in higher regard for its ancient pedigree and the difficulty of gaining access to it, pepper came to be a major commodity that would eventually come to determine what group would dominate European markets. Under Augustus, the pepper route between India and Egypt was established so that Romans would not depend on the Arab monopoly on the spice (Miller, 1969). By the Middle Ages, pepper had become the most popular spice, frequently sought by the middle class as larger supplies of it became available. Pepper was distinguished by shape, color, and origin. Regardless of color and species, peppers were believed to be medicinal because of their warming qualities; Hippocrates described pepper as an antidote for poisons. A popular remedy for cold humors or respiratory problems during the medieval period included pepper, ginger, cloves, and wine.

Long pepper (*Piper longum*) from Southeast Asia circulated in Europe before black pepper became available. The flower resembles a cone, from which tiny clustered berries are harvested. During the Roman Empire, this pungent pepper was valued more highly than other peppers. Dried long pepper cones were thought to be useful for respiratory ailments in both Ayurvedic and Unani medicine, while the root was thought to be useful as an appetite stimulant. Black pepper (*Piper nigrum*) consists of the dried berry and comes from many different sites across Southeast Asia and India. Peppercorns can be black, green, white, or red/pink. "White pepper" is a peppercorn with its outer layer removed. Black pepper came to dominate European tastes in the Middle Ages. Peppercorns were frequently used as currency to pay tax, rent, tribute, ransom, and salaries.

Red pepper is the fruit of the capsicum genus. While black pepper was immensely popular for centuries and continues to be ubiquitous, capsicum has a near-cultlike following today and is celebrated in regional festivals, especially in Mexico and the southwestern United States. This New World pepper is known by a number of names: cayenne, chili, paprika, and pimento, among others. There are many varieties (*Capsicum annum, C. baccatum, C. chinense, C. frutense, and C. pubescens*) ranging from sweet to hot. The more pungent versions are considered to be powerful stimulants for the digestive system and are also useful in aiding circulation. Plasters are adhesive bandages treated with herbal remedies; one type of Asian plaster contains cayenne. (A version of this plaster is currently available in U.S. drugstores.) Cayenne is believed to have antibiotic as well as anesthetic qualities. Consumed fresh or in dried form, capsicum is believed to be a tonic that aids metabolism. Healers in some Native American tribal societies used chilies to facilitate healing visions.

TODAY'S SPICES

By the twentieth century, spices were classified as aromatic substances used as food seasonings, as well as ingredients in drugs, candies, and cordials. A 1915 U.S. reference book on spices intended for the "inspector, chemist, manufacturer, buyer, salesman" indicates various classifications in the spice industry (Jank, 1915). Inspectors ascertain acceptable qualities and quantities of spices in industrial foodways. This was a response to the nineteenth-century promotion of tonics and patent medicines that were advertised as cure-alls for almost any ailment, including indigestion, headache, dyspepsia, fevers, loss of appetite, and loss of energy. Many patent medicines had high alcohol content, ranging up to 40 percent. Spices were categorized according to pungency, volatile oils, use, and preservative qualities.

The legacy of spices is most evident in various cuisines along the trade routes, as well as in remote areas far from centers of

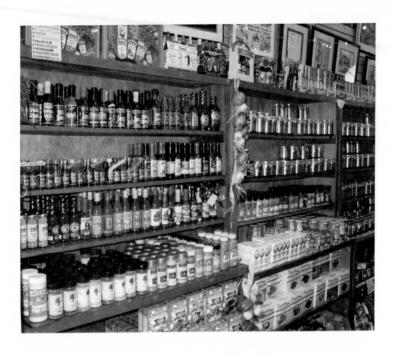

Hot sauces in French market, New Orleans, 2005

commerce. Many dishes are not complete without specific spices in combination with particular ingredients. Spice markets throughout Europe, particularly in Amsterdam and Paris, are contemporary "museums" for studying the history of the colonial exportation of spices from Asia. Grocers in France were originally referred to as *épiciers*, spice merchants. These markets handsomely display herbs and spices from various Asian sites and exotic tropical islands. The Grande Épicerie in Le Bon Marché (a department store) in Paris continues this tradition. Whole aisles are devoted to different salts, peppers, vanilla beans, cocoa, tea, and herbs in elaborate display.

Today's spice rack includes many spices in powder form, so that they can be sprinkled onto food. Audre Lorde's memory of her mother blending spices with a mortar and pestle demonstrates the more traditional way to process spices. Some spice cakes and breads include many kinds of spices, ranging from ginger, nutmeg, mace, and cinnamon to cloves.

A Healthy, Long Life

Longevity is a particular ideal that can be found across many cultures. In both historical and contemporary times, specific diets and food practices have this goal in mind. Why are certain foods thought to be conducive to long life? Daoist and other traditions addressed longevity as a goal and ascribed specific properties to certain foods and spices. Longevity meant more than an extended length of life; it also meant living free of disease and illness. Research on centenarians from various regions offers another approach to the study of longevity. Ironically, many diets with the aim of long life involve either abstinence or restricted caloric intake.

Across many cultures, drinking and eating are often begun or punctuated with wishes for health and long life. The deep-seated obsession with longevity has a long tradition in Chinese culture. Wishes and greetings for the Chinese New Year frequently include salutations for health, wealth, and long life. Long-lived sages and immortal figures are found in a broad spectrum of Chinese popular culture. Sun Simiao was an early physician who after his 101-year life was frequently referred to as the god of medicine. The monkey king is a folkloric figure who was reputed to have gained immortality by illicitly consuming peaches intended for sages. His exploits are detailed in one of the four great classic novels of Chinese literature, *Journey to the West*.

This fascination with immortality and longevity was a common theme in Daoist spiritual practice. To live to the age of 60, finishing five 12-year cycles, was considered to be the ideal. Daoist adepts were reputed to live twice as long, to the age of 120 or longer, well beyond normal human life expectancy in ancient China. Health was a treasure to be maintained and nourished through following the Dao with daily regimens of breathing, eating, and being in the world. To become ill or succumb to disease was to lose the way. Longevity was not the sole goal of Daoism; rather, it was part of the way. The earliest Chinese medical literature incorporated Daoist herbal knowledge and notions of qi energy. Medicinal herbs continue to be deemed valuable according to their ability to promote longer life and well-being.

The relation between diet and spiritual practice can be found in many religious traditions. The term "ascetic" is derived from Greek *askesis*, referring to exercise or training, and from *asketikos*, meaning industrious and athletic. Ascetics in both Christian and Buddhist traditions were known for their renouncement of material or worldly comforts, and they practiced self-denial to demonstrate their devotion. For example, fasting was used to purify the body in preparation for a better spiritual life. Longevity in such cases emphasized a spiritual life over a physical one, and the holistic emphasis on physical well-being as part of a spiritual path enabled a preventive approach to disease and suffering. Because many of the diseases of the ancient world were diet-related, an emphasis on humoral balance promoted wellness by situating a person's health within a broader spectrum of environmental and dietary factors.

The desire for longevity can be traced across many cultures. Legends of the fountain of youth, where taking the waters could help shed years of aging, inspired Spanish explorer Ponce de Leon to seek this site, known as Bimini, in the Bahamas. Lucas Cranach the Elder's sixteenth-century painting depicts the fountain of youth as a pool in which elderly pilgrims entered and departed as their youthful selves. Desires for longer lives unencumbered by illness have led many to seek practices promoting anti-aging. Diets in particular have been a focus for research on longevity.

CENTENARIAN DIETS

In 1973, *National Geographic* published a story on the oldest living humans, inhabitants of the Caucasus region of the former Soviet Union. Over many generations, they were reported to live well into their 100s. These centenarians were mostly nomadic herders living on simple diets consisting primarily of yogurt, garlic, seasonal foods, and occasionally meat. They commonly practiced herbal medicine. In Azerbaijian, an elderly centenarian, Shirali Muslimov, was supposed to have lived to the age of 168 and to have had five generations of descendants. In the absence of accurate records, gerontologists question the actual ages these people have claimed, but these stories nonetheless have captured the public imagination.

Several other regions of the world, including the Hunza Valley of Pakistan and Vilcabamba in Ecuador, have been reported to have large numbers of people living for a century or more. More centenarians have recently been reported in Okinawa, and the number seems to be growing in China and the United States. Approximately 90 percent of centenarians are women, regardless of region. Jeanne Calment, a Frenchwoman, died in 1997 at the documented age of 122.

While genetics play a key role in determining the length and quality of life, diet, which can promote or exacerbate ill health, is also a critical factor. Not surprisingly, many longevity regimens entail fasting or caloric restriction. Traditional medical knowledge consistently addresses how inappropriate consumption of food leads to imbalances that can damage internal organs and circulation. Biomedical practitioners concur on the importance of nutrition in health. Diets that contain excessive fat and sugar are not deemed healthy. The 2004 documentary *Supersize Me* demonstrated the effect of an exclusively fast-food diet eaten over 30 days. Not only did the filmmaker gain weight, he also suffered ill effects, ranging from headaches and high blood pressure to exhaustion. According to the Robert Woods Johnson Foundation, over 125 million Americans have a chronic health condition (lasting over a year) such as diabetes, cancer, or heart disease, and 60 million have more than one. This number is expected to climb as younger persons under the age of 45 and more children become diagnosed with chronic illnesses, further increasing the cost of health care. Many chronic conditions can be alleviated or exacerbated by diet.

The Hunza Valley, in the Himalayan range of northern Pakistan adjoining western China, has sometimes been said to be the inspiration for Shangri-La, an edenic lost paradise. The valley, also known as the land of vitality, is home to one of the largest concentrations of geriatric citizens in good health. In 1927, British researcher Sir Robert McCarrison conducted a study of the Hunzakut diet. Rats were fed unprocessed foods, mostly locally grown fruits and vegetables, milk products, whole grains, and little meat. After 27 months, the rats were found to have no morbid symptoms of disease. They seemed to thrive longer than two comparative groups, one fed the diet of a poorer region in India, and the other fed the diet of the British working class—tea with sugar, jam, margarine, and canned meats. Since this study, researchers in the latter half of the twentieth century have suggested that both the apricots of this region and the mineral content of the water may have contributed to the longevity of Hunza Valley inhabitants. Not surprisingly, Hunza water and apricot oil are currently promoted to increase longevity.

Okinawa is another region known for its growing number of elderly inhabitants. Okinawans eat a simple diet of unprocessed seasonal fruits and vegetables with soy, fish, and occasionally meat. Obesity, cancer, heart disease, stroke, senility, and dementia, conditions usually associated with old age, are relatively rare among Okinawans. Instead, the Okinawans' plant-based diet and plenty of exercise, among many other contributing factors such as genetics, ensure that the elderly in this region are healthy well into their 90s.

Nutritionists and scientists continue research on centenarians and their diets, looking for clues that might promote long life. It is clear there is a common thread among these disparate regions: a simple diet combined with daily activity ensures healthy living. Cultural practices that prescribe meal times, appropriate foods, and the amounts of food consumed are equally important. Diets must be considered in context. It is not possible, for example, to replicate the Hunza Valley diet elsewhere without consideration of the diet in a broader spectrum in which social contexts of consumption and activity contribute to longevity. Long life may be in the genes, but it is also located in cultural systems of knowledge and practice.

LONGEVITY HERBS: GINSENG, GINGKO, AND RHUBARB

The search for long life has also focused on specific foods and herbs. Ginseng, used in ancient times, is the herb most commonly associated with longevity. The root is believed

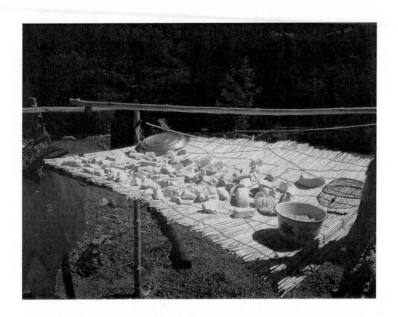

Homemade cheese from Kazakh nomads in Altai Mountains,
Xinjiang, 2003 (photo courtesy Dr. Dru C. Gladney)

to contain tonic qualities of the five elements, which can be imparted through consumption. There are several varieties of ginseng—Chinese, Korean, American, and Vietnamese—each of which is considered to have different therapeutic properties. Overall, the ginsenosides are deemed to have many health-promoting properties, including analgesic, anti-inflammatory, anticonvulsive, digestive, and calming. Daoists considered ginseng to be the king of herbs that could extend life. The herb is mostly acquired in root form, which may then be sliced, ground, or distilled. Most Chinese medical preparations include ginseng as a tea or as a liquid, like chicken broth. Ginseng extract can be consumed in liquid form as a dietary supplement.

Ginkgo is another plant frequently associated with longevity in Asia. Ginkgo seeds can be roasted alone or combined with other foods as a tonic. The seeds were viewed in Chinese tradition as precious delicacies and were offered to the emperor, as well as honored guests. On a summer stroll through the Temple of Heaven (Tiantan) in Beijing, I noticed ginkgo trees that are several thousand years old. Medicinal uses of this herb abound; the fan-shaped leaves can be used in several ways. Brewed as a tea, ginkgo is deemed useful for respiratory and circulatory problems. In powder form and inhaled form, this herb is useful for ear, nose, and throat problems. The boiled leaves may also be used as a plaster for wounds or for chilblains, itchy skin inflammations that are the result of poor circulation and exposure to cold. Because ginkgo increases blood flow to the brain, enhances overall circulation, and is believed to increase kidney yang sexual energy, this medicinal herb has been closely tied to longevity and the good life.[2]

While ginseng and ginkgo are known to be longevity herbs, rhubarb is less well known as an aid to longer life. Rhubarb today is often thought of only as a filler in fruit pies. The story of rhubarb as part of the Western diet begins with the Mongols on the Silk Road (Foust, 1992). Native to Mongolia, Siberia, Tibet, the Himalayas, and the Altai mountains, rhubarb grows in the wild as a low-lying shrub. There are several varieties, including *Rheum palmatum*, *R. raponticum*, *R. officiale*, *R. tanguticum*, *R. webbianum*, and *R. emodi*. The medical species is quite different from the domesticated garden rhubarb. The leaves, stalks, and roots of *R. palmatum* are used according to the desired effect. High in oxalic acid, the leaves are boiled and used as a purgative. The roots are rhizomes that reproduce. The hearty plant survives at high altitudes and in cold weather. Mongol troops reportedly carried rhubarb roots with them on their military campaigns for medicinal purposes—primarily for its digestive, laxative, and diuretic properties. Marco Polo is credited

ROASTED GINKGO NUTS

The leaves, seeds, and roots of the gingko biloba tree have many uses in Chinese medicine. They are believed to promote memory and enhance circulation, and they are especially important for cardiovascular health. I first tasted roasted ginkgo nuts at the end of a banquet in a private home in Cambridge, Massachusetts. The roasted seeds have a delicate flavor and can be used in combination with other foods in Chinese medicinal recipes like chicken with shitake mushrooms. Raw seeds can be quite toxic, and children should not consume them.

with bringing knowledge of this unusual plant to Europe. On the Silk Road, rhubarb was traded along with cassia and ceramics.

During the nineteenth and early twentieth centuries, rhubarb became a culinary fashion after the Dutch East India Company traded it as a rare commodity. English people and Germans in particular grew to like this sour-tasting plant and developed soups and desserts with rhubarb, especially after the sugar industry made sweeteners readily available. Under Peter the Great, there was a state monopoly on rhubarb, which was later broken up by Catherine the Great. During the Qing Dynasty (1759–1790), exports of rhubarb to Russia and other foreign countries were explicitly banned. Domesticated rhubarb is mostly eaten for its stalks, while the leaves are deemed toxic and thus thrown away. Today body-building websites promote rhubarb as a dietary supplement for weight loss and fat burning.

LONGEVITY IN PILL FORM

The allure of longevity can also be found in contemporary dietary supplements that are promoted as ways to increase energy and slow down the effects of aging. As life expectancy has improved in many countries with increasingly large elderly populations, the anti-aging industry, made up of small pharmaceutical firms, cosmetic companies, venture capitalists, and food supplement firms, have turned to longevity and anti-aging as a growth industry. In the United States in the twentieth century, life expectancy increased from 47 to 77 years. The baby boomer generation in their 50s and 60s will number 76 million in this decade.[3] Like the diet industry, the anti-aging industry is big business, generating profits in the range of $45 billion overall per year. Synthetic hormones and enzymes to redress mental decline and physical aging are just parts of the new product line.

Theories of aging over the past two decades have focused on environmental factors and on cellular processes that lead to aging. Earlier theories have addressed the role of free radicals and oxidation in wearing down the body. More recent scientific focus is concerned with cellular models of aging. An aging cell tends to have mitochondria that are less responsive in normal functions. Biopharmaceutical firms have developed new supplements that supposedly slow down the effects of aging by replenishing the mitochondria.

The anti-aging industry promotes a particular image of longevity that is reduced to biomechanical processes at the cellular level. Such discourse focuses on longevity as an individual body's battle against aging rather than considering aging in a broader social and historical context. In an era when care of the self comprises a vast industry, healing through nutrition and healthy diets may seem too low-tech or slow. Gaining broader cultural knowledge of medicinal foods may offer alternatives to anti-aging discourse in which bodies are subject to biomechanical processes. Traditional systems of medicine offered insights based on observation of the subtle interactions of food and environment of human bodies. We can greatly influence our well-being through diet and nutritional knowledge, not just consuming dietary supplements. Longevity is not guaranteed, but the possibility of accessible self-managed care on a daily basis through attention to one's food can enhance the quality of one's life.

CHAPTER TWO

Dietary Prescriptions and Comfort Foods

Dietary standards change over time and reflect shifting views concerning nutrition and well-being. In many social groups and cultural systems, one's identity or group membership is determined by dietary practices. The transformation of certain medicines and food can be found not only in the North American or European context but also in developing nations with new consumers who participate in a globalized diet of industrial foods. The current "epidemic" of obesity in North America can also be seen among elites in developing nations. Even though foods may still be viewed as medicinal in the contemporary moment, industrial foodways, the pharmaceutical industry, the fast food industry, and increasingly sedentary lifestyles have significantly affected nutrition and the uses of healing foods. As theories of diet and nutrition are constantly being revised, health risks and notions of food excess or nutritional deficiency may change over generations. In the examination of diet as a cultural practice, I address how dietary prescriptions evolve during different periods in which knowledge of nutrition changes. In particular, I address how salt and sugar have been valorized or vilified in various dietary prescriptions. I also consider fat: how some foodways still consider it an invaluable source of heat or energy, while in North American discourse trans fat has become a dietary evil.

In chapter 1, I examine how food and medicine were considered inseparable in the path to well-being and longevity. Longevity was in ancient times and continues to be an ideal. What constitutes good food or medicine in the promotion of long life or self-care? Is what is good for the self also good for the body? A new category, comfort food, raises important questions about food, self, and identity. Satiation, feeling satisfied by food, and enjoyment of taste are particular cultural values that are worth exploring in the relationship between food and medicine. Chinese herbal medicine has been frequently described as bitter tasting. Similarly, pills and tonics without additional flavoring can be described as unappetizing, often having a bitter aftertaste. Does sweetness, or its cultural equivalences, make everything better?

Dieting and Everyday Life

The work of anthropology is most frequently associated with other cultures and places. The lessons learned from other cultures offer a critical tool of reflection on one's own society and cultural practices. Defamiliarization, in which the unfamiliar becomes understandable while what was once familiar becomes exotic, offers a useful way to frame dietary practices as a cultural form. I once asked a Chinese colleague who had come to visit the United States for the first time what his impressions had been. He immediately named the highway system, the clean air—and widespread obesity. He claimed that he had never seen so many overweight people. The large portions of food in a single serving were unfamiliar to him. Obesity, in fact, is quickly becoming a global concern. China, for instance, recently reported higher rates of obesity among children and urban dwellers due to changes in consumption and increasingly sedentary ways of living.

Anthropology focuses on rituals that offer solidarity and help create identities. Attention to daily life also offers powerful ways to view our social worlds and the personal meanings we give to our lives. In this view, diets, or what and how we consume, tell us much about the formation of identity and being in the world.

People of many ages and backgrounds follow diets in which either calories or food groups are restricted. Diets in calorie- and fat-obsessed North American culture are understood as the control of food intake to reduce weight. Television and print media frequently include advertisements featuring personal testimonials to the effectiveness of a particular dietary regimen, which, ironically, run alongside advertisements for fast food, alcohol, and soft drinks. Conversations over meals often center on dietary regimens or on the ingredients of prepared foods. Different dieting trends or fads may emphasize particular food categories such as protein and carbohydrates or recommend the restriction, or even elimination, of items such as sugar and fat. Dieting has quickly been adapted as a form of defining the self, as well as shaping the body. Diets vary widely, and despite the different forms they take, behind most of them is the common goal of health. Analyzing diets as ritual forms that shape the self offers insights to how food consumption, solidarity, and selfhood are intimately linked. Though dieting to lose weight or as a form of restriction has been documented for several centuries, the shift from concerns for longevity and freedom from illness to widespread concerns about obesity and the near-obsession with thinness appears to mark contemporary consumer culture.

The story of dieting in North America reflects ongoing social and spiritual movements. Dieting in this country has ties to religious movements that flourished in the late nineteenth century. Before the rise of the dieting industry, diet was considered to be part of one's overall health regimen, which was linked to philosophies of spirituality and daily life. Many nineteenth-century temperance and social movements advocated vegetarianism, and they restricted consumption of certain foods to promote a higher degree of morality. Victorian health practices and diet therapies intended to promote healthy living required abstaining from foods or stimulants that were believed to encourage overeating and sexual appetites. Meals consisting of vegetables and grains, especially whole wheat, became widespread during this period, as did many health foods and breakfast cereals.

Graham crackers were promoted by Sylvester Graham, a Presbyterian minister based in New England who believed that consuming high-fiber wheat flour promoted a healthier and moral life. The normal diet of his era was high in animal fats and refined grains, which he considered stimulants that promoted excessive sexual urges. While Graham's preachings were considered eccentric in his time, they seem to have anticipated the contemporary linkage between modified consumption and high-fiber intake as a means to better health. Ironically, today's graham crackers contain sugar as a key ingredient, while his were made sweet through honey and molasses.

Today's breakfast cereals also share links to nineteenth-century temperance beliefs and health practices. Sanitariums were common during this period, and the rest cure was deemed the best way to treat neurasthenia, a complex of symptoms described as nervousness and anxiety. Perhaps the most well known of these institutions was the Battle Creek Sanitarium in Michigan, established by the Seventh-Day Adventists, who also advocated a moderate diet of vegetarianism and whole grains. As director, Dr. John Harvey Kellogg formulated granola and corn flakes to serve to patrons who stayed at the sanitarium. With his brother, he later packaged these foods and incorporated the Kellogg's cereal company. C. W. Post, the inventor of Grape Nuts cereal and Postum, a coffee substitute, developed his products after a long stay in the sanitarium. Today's sugary children's cereals, hawked during Saturday morning cartoons, are a far cry from the breakfast cereals of the late nineteenth century.

The story of Quaker Oats offers insight into the emergence of food companies in the late nineteenth century. Before they were processed, oats were sold in bulk form. Several milling companies began to sell processed oats, incorporating them under one name, the American Cereal Company. The emblem of a male Quaker on the box was meant to symbolize purity and wholesomeness. That image has persisted, Quaker Oats being one of the oldest brands associated with breakfast cereals.

The popularity of special diets coincided with the broader use of patent medicines, drugs whose names or container forms were trademarked. The ingredients themselves were less likely to be patented, and homemade versions of such remedies were well known. Patent medicines enjoyed widespread popularity around the turn of the twentieth century (Dupuis, 2007). Print media from this period frequently included advertisements with claims of miraculous cures from elixirs that contained mostly alcohol, vegetable extracts, and some sedative or stimulant such as opium, morphine, caffeine, or cocaine.

Dieting and the Body Politic

Prescriptions about food consumption, whether of intake, restriction, or avoidance, are situated cultural practices that reflect a great deal about belief systems. Eating particular foods, restricting others, or going on fasts continue to form a critical part of daily life for the spiritual practices of many faiths. The Bible holds many prescriptions for food consumption, including definitions of purity and pollution. Mary Douglas's analysis of the "Abominations of Leviticus" indicates how those guidelines create meaning and shape material practices such as the preparation and consumption of food (1984). Jewish kashrut or dietary laws continue in the present moment as categories of kosher or cleanliness that entail certification of proper slaughter or preparation in which forbidden animals such as shellfish or rabbit are not included. Muslim dietary laws also have strict categories of halal or cleanliness that include proper slaughter and restrictions on certain animal flesh such as pork. Buddhist dietary practices consider the slaughter of animals to be unclean; hence, Buddhists of certain sects do not consume meat. Ironically, vegetarian restaurants in Asia have extensive menus filled with mock duck, goose, beef, and chicken dishes that contain gluten and soy as meat substitutes.

During the early twentieth century, the U.S. government regularly issued dietary prescriptions addressing caloric intake to domestic consumers. Marion Nestle's examination of this century in *Food Politics* identifies two distinct stages—pre–

World War II and post–World War I—in which the federal government articulated very different advice about eating (2002). The early half of the twentieth century was characterized by an "eat more" policy to combat poverty and hunger. This shifted in the second half of the century to an "eat less" approach, as scientific studies linked chronic and long-term health conditions such as heart disease and diabetes to diet. Addressing dietary policy offers insight into how governments view the bodies of citizens, especially healthy bodies, as critical to the well-being of the nation. Healthy bodies make for a strong nation.

The association between diets and nationalism is longstanding. Early Greek writings in the Hippocratic Corpus associate the body of citizens as representative of the body politic. Olympian games in ancient Greece, as well as today, offer displays of able and fit bodies. What goes into the making of such near-perfect bodies has included not only physical regimens of training but also dietary practices associated with fitness. National policies on health, fitness, and dietary prescriptions can be found in many countries. During the Republican era in mainland China, intense emphasis on the New Life campaign focused on the family, especially young children and women (Glosser, 2003). During the 1930s, the consumption of milk in particular was heavily emphasized for Chinese children and nursing mothers. During World War II, Great Britain and other Allied nations offered suggestions for patriotic consumption of local or independently produced goods and the renunciation of goods that were considered to support enemy economies. The political attempt to rename French fries "freedom fries" in 2003, when anti-French sentiment in the United States ran high, also illustrates the link between consumption and nationalism.

Dieting has been included in a range of social practices among many cultlike groups. Indeed, many cults and religious sects have included specific diets to create social identities and maintain boundaries between those who are included, or not, among followers. Fasting is also encouraged by many spiritual groups to promote bodily and spiritual cleansing.

The culture of dieting thus has a particular history in the United States with links to temperance movements, food companies in the industrial age, and spiritual beliefs. Philosophies of dieting in the early twentieth century were tied to moral discourses of well-being as an integral part of spiritual life. Consumption of polluting substances was believed to lead to gluttony and other immoral behavior. In what follows, we turn to the ways in which dieting is linked to a range of health concerns such as obesity, diabetes, and heart disease. The transformation from dieting as a reflection of morality into dieting as part of nutritional knowledge and biomedical practice reveals the ways in which science and medicine have structured meanings of dietary prescriptions. In particular, salt, sugar, and fat have been valorized or vilified in various dietary prescriptions.

Salt

Growing up in Louisiana, I often saw people adding salt to their watermelon. Rather than making the fruit taste saltier, consumers claimed that the contrast enhanced the sweetness of the melon. Perhaps more than spices, salt is regularly added to foods either during cooking and before eating or in prepared foods. On many American tables, especially in restaurants, salt and pepper shakers are ubiquitous. Like pepper, salt has a long history of travel and trade. It is a mineral rather than a plant-based spice.

The story of salt is also a story of industrialization. Several recent texts document the history of salt and its cultural contexts (Laszlo, 2001; Kurlansky, 2002b). Whereas spices traveled from Asia to Europe in a unidirectional flow, salt could be found in many places. Salt could be harvested from the sea using salt flats or pans. Salt, called "white gold," could also be found in the ground, the product of elaborate salt mines (Laszlo, 2001). Salt enabled the preservation and travel of many food items such as fish, meat, and vegetables. Whereas spices initially reflected exclusivity, salt became ubiquitous for meanings of worth. The term "salary" is derived from the Latin *salarium*, Roman soldiers receiving salt rations for their wages. Salt in various European languages came to reflect certain notions of character and ability.

Salt transforms the flavor of foods. While it is not addictive, many people claim to crave salty foods. It is an essential part of the human diet, helping to maintain bodily fluids and functions. There is some controversy about the effects of salt on blood pressure. While excess sodium has been proven to be detrimental to health because it raises blood pressure, the salt industry has been quick to point out that salt does not necessarily have that effect on everyone.[1] Rather, they argue, overall food quality has a greater impact than salt content on well-being. In 1995, the Food and Drug Administration (FDA) announced, on the recommendation of the National Research Council, that the recommended minimum intake of sodium be 500 mg daily value (DV) with an upper limit of 2400 mg.[2] Though the council recommended an even lower intake, 1800 mg DV, the average sodium consumption is closer to 6000 mg DV.

In the United States today, less attention is paid to the established ill effects of too much salt than to identifying hidden salts in processed foods. Such hidden salts are usually in the form of monosodium glutamate or sodium bicarbonate. The majority of soft drinks, packaged meats, and sweets have a high sodium content. The linkage between salts and medicine is very important. Salts not only are produced for daily consumption but also are necessary in the production of pharmaceutical drugs and the chemical industry. The past decade has seen a revival of interest in handcrafted and harvested sea salts rather than industrially processed salt.

Sugar

Sweetness comes in many forms. There are multiple forms of sugar, including sucrose, glucose, fructose, lactose, galactose, and maltose. Sucrose, or table sugar, is the most commonly known, a combination of glucose and fructose. However, many naturally occurring sugars are found in fruits, vegetables, and milk. The desire for sweetness is not limited to humans. Physical anthropologists who work with primates have documented these animals' extensive searches for fermented fruit and other foods with higher sugar content even when other nutrient sources are readily available (Dominy, 2004).

Honey has inspired long journeys, often risking dangerous forays to acquire it. Long before sugar, honey was widely regarded as the nectar of gods and a key to good health. In addition to several sugars, honey also contains enzymes, antibiotics, minerals, acids, and vitamins. Legend and folklore around honey's innate medicinal qualities and its promotion of longevity are found in all ancient civilizations, including Chinese,

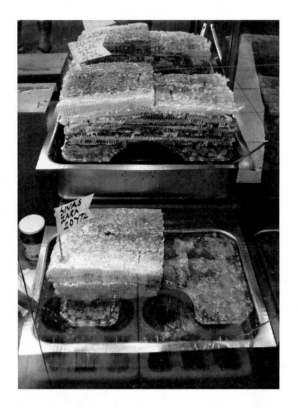

Raw honey in Egyptian spice market, Istanbul, 2006

Egyptian, Mayan, Greek, and Roman. Honey was regularly used as a preservative. Napoleon's body was encased in a vat of honey before it was returned to Paris from the isle of St. Helena. The concentrated nectar of flowers, wildflower honey in particular is regarded as especially medicinal and useful for stimulation of the immune system against allergies, viruses, fungi, infections, and inflammation.

The legendary qualities associated with honey easily transferred to sugar. Sugar from cane in unrefined forms was used as a sweetener in India, China, and Persia even before the

Crusades. The nursery rhyme "sugar and spice and every-thing nice" positions sugar in the good life. Sugar was sweet, of course, and also thought to be medicinal. Sugar can take different forms: as crystal, liquid, syrup, and refined grains, as well as powder. Vegetable sources of sugar include cane and beets. During the Renaissance, sugar was viewed as a spice and was included in the preparations of savory foods, not just pas-tries or candies (Mintz, 1986).

The association of sugar with medicine was further linked when apothecaries created various remedies that included sugar. The continued inclusion of sugar in medicine reflects the continuum that exists between food and medicine. Even today, many medicinal syrups, tonics, and pills include sugar or a sugar substitute to camouflage any bitter aftertaste. Con-temporary double-blind clinical trials still often use sugar pills as placebos.

Concern for sugar consumption and its link to obesity led to the chemical production of such low-calorie sweeteners as sac-charine and aspartame. Saccharine was widely consumed until it was linked to high cancer rates, which led to the search for other sweeteners. According to the official Nutrasweet web-site, aspartame is included in over 5,000 foods and beverages.[3] There is much controversy about the uses of these artificial sweeteners and their links to a number of illnesses. The desire for sweetness, nevertheless, drives the inclusion of these in-gredients in many soft drinks and processed foods. In the past decade, attention has been paid to a natural sweetener derived from the leaves of *Stevia rebaudiana*, a South American plant known commonly as "stevia." My first encounter with this herb was in a Santa Cruz medicinal garden, where a student studying herbal medicine gave me a taste of its leaves. Expect-ing a bitter leafy flavor, I tasted instead a surprising sweetness that released with each chew. Reported to be low in calories but several hundred times sweeter than sugar, the herb is sold in health food stores as a dietary supplement because of FDA restrictions.[4] The herb is now available in powder form and is increasingly marketed to people, such as diabetics, seeking nonsugar alternatives.

While sugar was highly regarded for flavoring and for its medicinal qualities when it was first introduced into the West, by the late twentieth century sugar was linked to health concerns such as obesity, diabetes, and hyperactivity. Members of the biomedical establishment have repeatedly denied any linkage of sugar to hyperactivity or attention deficit disorder. Nonetheless, sugar's dangers have long eclipsed its earlier associations with goodness.

Fat

My godmother in Beijing makes a delicious winter dish of braised pork where a rump roast with one to two inches of pure fat is simmered slowly with soy sauce and sugar. In the final assemblage, the sugar is caramelized and the sauce poured over the roast such that the fat melts in one's mouth. As an American who spent a decade in body-conscious California, it was hard to get over the fact that I was basically consuming pure animal fat. Yet the loving attention my godmother gave to making this dish and its rich flavor overcame my concerns that eating it would be deemed unhealthy, hence taboo, by Californian standards.

The concern or near-obsession with fat in North America is not unwarranted as obesity has increased significantly in the United States, to the extent that the Centers for Disease

Control and Prevention (CDC) released studies in 1999 and announced that this public health concern would lead to higher death rates than the former number-one concern, coronary heart disease. Obesity is considered to be epidemic among children and adolescents in the country, with up to 30 percent identified as clinically obese (Oliver, 2006). Defined as having a body mass index of over 30, obesity has doubled in the past two decades for adults and children, while obese adolescents have tripled in number. In one year alone, 1998, obesity jumped 6 percent.

Numerous factors are associated with obesity: increasingly sedentary habits, genetic predisposition, and poor nutrition, among them. The effect of chronic health conditions and higher mortality at a younger age has been cause for great concern among nutritionists and policy makers. Increased television watching, video game playing, and computer use are also blamed. The postindustrial television era has greatly influenced American popular culture, and food is not exempt.

Researchers have noted that it may not necessarily be the increased hours that people spend watching TV that is the problem, but also that a lot of this time is spent watching commercials for fast foods, snacks, and beverages. Second only to automobile advertising, the food and beverage industry in the United States spends most of their dollars on prime-time television advertising. In children's television programming, food ads account for 50 percent of commercial time; every five minutes, there is a food-related ad (Kotz and Story, 1994). Young children recognize the latest snacks or prepared meals from watching TV and may clamor for them on family shopping trips, which has a significant economic impact.

It is helpful to consider the distinctions between dietary fat and body fat. One-third of the average American adult diet contains fat. Many essential fatty acids are actually an important source of concentrated energy. Dietary fat, however, is quite different from body fat, in which stores of fat cells are held in adipose tissue in the body. Subcutaneous body fat is one measurement of obesity, but visceral fat, or fat surrounding internal organs beneath subcutaneous layers, is considered much more harmful and lately has been of more concern than before.

It is also important to consider the role of food processing in the production of dietary fat. Fats come in three categories: saturated, unsaturated, and polyunsaturated. Of the three, the first is considered to be the unhealthiest, producing increased cholesterol, which affects the healthy functioning of the heart. When oils become partly hydrogenated (or hardened), many form trans fat, which has the same effect as saturated fats on cholesterol. This has become the new element of concern in processed foods. The food industry uses trans fat to extend shelf life, increase texture, and reduce costs. Until 2006, information about trans fats was not required on nutrition information panels. Many processed foods such as potato chips now say on their packaging "zero trans fat," which seems to indicate no fat, when in fact they still contain a significant amount of dietary fat.

Regardless of where excess fat or calories comes from, the concern for obesity has led some local communities to intervene in primary schools over diet. American chef and restaurateur Alice Waters has forged links between schools and farmers' markets and encouraged gardens run by schools to bring fresh produce into school cafeterias. Teaching young children and adolescents how to choose healthier food options is a crucial step toward enabling the younger generation to avoid preventable disease.

Soft Drinks, Hard Currency

Beverages tend to be emphasized less commonly than solid food, but they are critically linked to concerns of diet and health. For instance, the consumption of soda several times a day has health consequences, and the substitution of a liquid diet supplement for a meal raises questions about what defines a proper meal and whether eating solids is a necessary component.

Beverages include coffee, tea, milk, mineral water, juice, smoothies, carbonated soft drinks, noncarbonated soft drinks, wine, beer, and hard liquor. Beverages were frequently included in rituals of ancient civilizations, as documented in written and pictorial sources. In ancient China, for instance, elaborate bronze vessels for the ritual drinking of wine date to the Shang Dynasty (2000 B.C.). Later, the ancient Greeks (200 B.C.) bestowed honors to Dionysius in rituals using wine. The Greek symposium was a banquet or drinking party where ideas and toasts were exchanged, as opposed to a formal meeting. Most cultures do have some form of indigenous liquor from fermented grains or vegetables that may be consumed outside of a ritual context (Holt, 2006). In medieval Europe, the average consumption of beer per person, including children, was 3 liters per day. Beer mash was consumed for breakfast in some parts of Europe. In Asia, a form of mash made from fermented rice can be consumed for breakfast or distilled further into rice wine or sake. In this section, I focus primarily on soft drinks and carbonated beverages that contain high-fructose corn syrup as a main ingredient as sweetener.

As beverages, the history and social worlds of coffee and tea, drinks that emerged worldwide with mercantile capitalism, have been extensively documented. Even milk, considered to be wholesome and pure, became prevalent only with the rise of the dairy industry (Dupuis, 2002). Less discussed are soft drinks, which have grown exponentially in the global market. Soft drinks, carbonated beverages that contain high-fructose corn syrup, among other ingredients, is big business and is generating new categories of medicinal drinks and liquid food. The cost of production is quite low since water, carbonation, and some flavoring are cheap; value is added through branding and advertisement. In the United States, soft drinks are the most popular form of liquid refreshment; more soft drinks are consumed than coffee, tea, and juice combined. The soft drink industry in this country is estimated at $58 billion.[5] In 1998, the average consumption of soft drinks was 56 gallons per person per year. In 2007, the market was estimated to grow by 5 percent each year. Not all soft drinks are the same. The cola wars of the 1980s and the 1990s ushered in the new "uncolas" of this decade, which seek a younger, hipper audience—such as bicyclists and snowboarders.[6]

Carbonated beverages stem from mineral waters, which, primarily in the form of healing baths, have long been considered to be therapeutic. European spas and resorts at natural springs came to include drinking the water as part of the therapeutic process. When the water in mineral baths was analyzed, scientists found carbonium, or carbon dioxide, as a source of the bubbles in natural springs. Soon after, scientists mastered the artificial production of effervescent bubbles. Pharmacists were the first sellers of carbonated water in the nineteenth century. The soda fountain could create carbonated drinks and sell them as medicinal (Tufts, 1895). Being a soda jerk could be difficult work, as the early machinery to produce carbonated water under high pressure included sulfuric acid. Since mineral water has an aftertaste, the first forms of carbonated water had added syrup or flavorings. Many pharmacists experimented with additives believed to have curative properties, such as birch bark or dandelions, which led to the invention of ginger ale, root beer, sarsaparilla, and lemon soda. The corner drugstore became a public space for social gathering. The soft drink industry began to reach consumers at home as well as on the road as bottling the drinks became possible. Vending machines, introduced in the 1920s, further popularized soft drinks.

The main ingredients of a carbonated beverage are some or all of the following: water, carbon dioxide, flavors, colors, caffeine, acids, preservatives, potassium, sodium, phosphorus, and sweeteners—whether high-fructose corn syrup; sucrose from sugar cane or beets; or diet sweeteners such as aspartame, saccharine, sucralose, and acesulfame K. Coca-Cola is said to have originally included coca derivatives, though the company disputes this. Dr. John Pemberton, a pharmacist based in Atlanta, made Coca-Cola syrup from a concoction of herbs, then mixed it with carbonated water and served it at a soda fountain. The drink since then has become emblematic of America and is a widely known brand around the world. A scholar of material culture, Daniel Miller, argues that viewing the soft drink industry offers insight not only into local tastes but also how regional tastes developed global markets (1995, 1998). For instance, when the beverage was first introduced to Chinese consumers in the 1980s, it was not called Coca-Cola, which meant "horse dung." They called it instead *Kekou Koule*, which means "pleasure for thirst and the mouth." China has a number of cola drinks such as *Tianfu* (heavenly) cola, which is popular for its suggested effects on digestion. Some consumers in Mexico claim that cola there is sweeter due to the use of cane sugar rather than corn syrup sweeteners. New cola mixtures introduce flavors such as cherry, lemon/lime, vanilla, and chocolate to reach new audiences.

The consumption of soft drinks as part of everyday life, particularly among young children, has been a cause for concern for nutritionists and medical personnel. Nutritionists have called soft drinks liquid candy, especially for young children and adolescents. Tooth decay, delayed bone development, obesity, and diabetes are some of the health issues associated with excessive soda consumption. Children in the twenty-first century drink more soda than ever. The ubiquity of vending machines in schools makes soft drinks more accessible (Nestle, 2002). In the age group of 6–11 years, 60 percent of boys and 70 percent of girls fall short of the recommended amounts of calcium in their dietary intake. Milk—even chocolate milk, which, though sweet, is preferable to soda—is promoted to younger consumers to address this problem, as well as to cut down on soda consumption (Lin and Ralston, 2003). However, carbonated beverages are hard to avoid, particularly in fast food venues. The linkage of sodas with hamburgers, hot dogs, fried chicken, and pizza facilitates a diet high in sugar, fat, and calories.

Excessive consumption even of diet sodas still raises health concerns. Promoters of diet drinks tend to emphasize that they taste great and satisfy thirst while having no sugar and thus no calories. Having it all without having to worry about calories or fat obscures the potential risk of sugar substitutes. Aspartame, a sugar substitute, is controversial because of its associations with a range of chronic disorders such as fibromyalgia, cramps, seizures, vertigo, and multiple sclerosis–like symptoms—not to mention cancer in laboratory rats.[7]

Recent trends in the beverage market include more health drinks, including water enhanced with supplements ranging from vitamins, herbal derivatives, protein, and even fiber. Energy drinks represent another key growth area and new category associated with today's youth culture. Energy drinks often include taurine, a sulfonic acid found in bile, or guarana, a Brazilian tropical berry. Both ingredients are believed to impute energy in combination with caffeine, sugar, and herbal supplements. New brands and labels for soft drink beverages include Pimpjuice and Bawls for the hip-hop market.

Dieting as Culture

In recent years the dieting industry has had $40 billion in overall revenue, and this was projected to rise up to $55 billion in 2008.[8] The many different ways of dieting reflect ongoing shifts in beliefs about food, dietary practice, and stratified consumption. Rather than thinking about dieting as a personal practice, it may be helpful to consider the social aspect of dieting as a part of culture as well. Many dieters find strength in numbers. The more social support for their dieting practices, the more successful adherence to their own regimens. Weight Watchers, a program to facilitate dieting goals in a social context, offers group support as a means of creating structure in dieting.

The Atkins Diet has received a widespread following among American dieters since the late 1990s. Seeking long-term weight loss, dieters are urged to consume more protein-based foods and decrease if not entirely eliminate carbohydrates and starches from their diet. Devout followers have proclaimed that they have had more success with losing weight faster than with any other diets. Critics of the diet tend to be proponents of well-rounded nutrition, and they don't believe that it is healthy to consume only protein. The Paleolithic Diet is another high-protein diet that became popular in the late twentieth century. Based on the notion that hunter/gatherers consumed mostly protein and gathered fruits or vegetables rather than cultivat-

WOLFBERRY (*LYCIUM BARBARUM*) SOUP

Ingredients: Broth made with chicken, water, rice wine, ginger, bamboo, mushrooms, scallions, wolfberries, and salt

Prepare broth with fresh chicken, water, rice wine, and sliced ginger root. Add sliced bamboo stems or shoots, mushrooms, scallions, and a handful of wolfberries. Add salt to taste.

Wolfberry tea

For wolfberry tea, put a teaspoonful of dried wolfberries in a large cup and add hot boiling water to steep.

In Chinese medicine, wolfberries are said to nourish two very important organs, the kidney and liver. The berries may be eaten in dried form like raisins, but caution should be exercised as overeating is considered to be "overheating."

Wolfberries are available in Chinese food stores and some health food stores.

ing grains, followers of this diet believe that human bodies are not evolutionarily well adapted to grain consumption. The fact that contemporary hunter/gatherer groups have comparatively lower rates of obesity, diabetes, and heart disease is also cited as reasons for the success of the Paleolithic Diet.

On the other end of the spectrum, another diet fad includes raw foods, based on the belief that uncooked foods retain the most nutrients. Its proponents believe that cooking not only alters taste, texture, and composition but also removes important vitamins. Fruitopians take the raw food movement one step further by only consuming food, mostly fruits, that they believe to have been made without the aid of industrial agriculture. Many more food fads and miracle diets abound. The majority of diet gurus require a complete change of life-style as well as a transformation in diet. For instance, the Mediterranean Diet advocates not only eating different food items but also eating at different times in different places, together with higher-quality food and consuming less of it.

Comfort Foods

The notion of food as comfort informs many advertisements for prepared meals that can be consumed in the comfort of one's home. Restaurants that specialize in simple, home-cooked fare also appeal to notions of comfort and convenience. As a genre of cooking, comfort foods have become further codified as cookbooks have appeared that specialize in homemade dishes. Why are chicken soup, macaroni and cheese, mashed potatoes, rice porridge, and so on considered comfort food? Though comfort foods may be classified as bad foods because many of them have excessive sugar, fat, carbohydrates, or sodium, on a symbolic front this category of foods is thought to be good for you. Psychologically, comfort foods may represent ties to one's homeland or ancestral background, memories of childhood, or notions of belonging.

A more compelling cultural framework to understand comfort food may be in terms of satiation rather than health. Health concerns like longevity require ascetic abstinence—a far cry from gluttony or excess. In many cultures, feasting performs the social function of creating solidarity. In some food cultures, excessive display and consumption have been critical for forging group identity. Roman food orgies, medieval feasts, and Native American potlatches were renowned for extensive gorging. Behind feasting and other excessive eating occasions is the desire to restore harmony to what may be out of balance. Comfort foods offer a different sense of well-being, one not necessarily tied to how healthy a food item is. Rather, how soothing a particular dish or foodway may be for a particular moment determines the comfort that food provides. Nostalgic gastronomy shapes tastes and preferences that offer powerful links to one's social practices of eating.

Recent studies suggest that in anxious moments, eating sugary and fatty foods can alleviate stress.[9] Heightened stress, registered by the adrenal gland, stimulates glutocortocoid production, which promotes a craving for fatty and sweet foods that quickly deliver high energy to the brain. Chronic stress may lead to overeating as a form of self-medication. Biomedical studies of comfort foods high in fat or sugar illustrate how desires for certain food items categorized as "bad" may in fact be based in self-preserving models of survival.

The sages and Daoist adepts mentioned earlier did not conceive of mental illness or stress as a separate category from physical health. Instead, various disorders that today could be categorized as manic, depressive, or stress-related were conceptualized in terms of humoral and elemental unbalance. Foods that nourished the body were deemed critical for restoring balance to both mind and body. Both concepts—longevity and comfort—suggest a desire for the good life. Notions of longevity as an ideal can be translated into desires for comfort. With comfort foods, however, the place and time of consumption are central to meanings of satiation.

By thinking of dieting in social terms as well as something an individual pursues, we can understand why dieting, so compelling for so many different reasons, most likely will continue to be Big Business. Dieting practices and prescriptions reflect ongoing beliefs about purity and identity, as well as shaping social relations. Dieting represents a critical juncture between food and medicine. Cultural norms of what constitutes a proper diet determine the amount of food consumed and whether or not a food is medicinal. While nineteenth-century notions of diet were tied to moral philosophies of living, twentieth-century notions became simultaneously linked to science and to forms of forging an individual identity. With increasingly sedentary habits and the rise of fast food, obesity has become an ongoing concern. Ironically, the dieting industry will continue to flourish as long as the advertising of food permeates daily life. As a food genre, comfort foods emerged during the late-twentieth-century postindustrial period as a nostalgic practice that nonetheless becomes part of stratified consumption.

PART TWO

Medicine as Food

CHAPTER THREE

Nutraceuticals and Functional Foods

During the 1990s new forms of medicinal food or combinations of food and medicine emerged. Researchers have found that certain elements of the foods consumed for health reasons can be extracted from various plants and put into pills or powders or combined with food items. These forms are called "nutraceuticals" (from "nutrition" and "pharmaceuticals") and are sometimes referred to as "functional foods": foods and drinks that have physiological effects that may help reduce chronic disease. Stephen DeFelice, founder of the Foundation for Innovation in Medicine, coined the term "nutraceutical" in 1979 as any food item deemed to have health benefits. In the past decade, the nutraceutical industry has developed to meet growing interest from consumers and health care professionals. Nutraceuticals introduce key questions about medicine as food. Are these super foods enhanced with fortified compounds or just dietary supplements in food form instead of pills? Though conventional food and medicine are considered to be separate categories, new technologies are enabling novel forms of eating and drinking one's way to health.

Nutraceuticals range from properties found in garlic and grapes to bioengineered foods that have isolated compounds or supplements. Food science scholars further elaborate: "Nutriceuticals are naturally-derived, bioactive (usually phytochemical) compounds that have health promoting, disease preventing or medicinal properties" (Lachance and Saba, 2002: 00). The category of enriched foods or medicines consumed in the form of food is a booming industry. Omega three–enriched eggs, vitamin-enriched drinks, and calcium supplements in the form of chocolate are all readily available in markets. Between food supplements and the pharmaceutical industry, nutraceuticals permeate daily life.

In ancient civilizations, dietary medicine viewed food and medicine as inseparable categories. For example, the Chinese imperial court under the Mongols ruled over a vast empire containing different peoples and food cultures. The wide range of foods served at court frequently included medicinal foods intended to extend the lifespan and quality of life for the ruler and his court. A cookbook submitted by the head chef in the thirteenth century documents the various recipes and foods served at court (Buell, Anderson, and Perry, 2000). In today's world, the boundaries are dissolving. In this chapter, I examine the blurred boundaries of medicine as food, comparing the claims of nutraceuticals with the associated benefits of nutrition. What are the consequences of treating food and medicine as separate categories—or not?

Functional foods are nutritious and also have specific health-promoting functions. For instance, garlic compounds are believed to be useful to lower hypertension, prevent cardiovascular heart disease, and even prevent or treat cancer. The association of lycopene, a carotenoid found in tomatoes, with the reduction of cancer cells has boosted the consumption of tomato-based foods. While the FDA has ruled that food manufacturers may not overtly promote a product as cancer-reducing, research on this topic continues to be funded by the food industry. Although the term "functional foods" is generally used to refer to unmodified foods, today, both genetically modified and vitamin-fortified foods are increasingly considered to be functional foods as well. The food industry tends to use the terms interchangeably; there is even a journal named *Functional Foods and Nutraceuticals*.

It can be argued that certain teas, tonics, and elixirs have long been used as medicine. Green teas, prepared by adding hot water to leaves of the *Camellia sinesis* plant or other herbs, were considered restorative and medicinal. Tonics were believed to have reviving qualities that tone and energize the body. Today, gin and tonic is a well-known cocktail, but in the nineteenth century, tonic water was derived from quinine and was consumed for its anti-malaria properties. Elixirs, nonalcoholic medicinal preparations usually in the form of syrups or beverages, hark back to Iraqi and Persian medical texts that were adapted by medieval apothecaries. Elixirs were prepared according to formulary instructions and consumed as cordials or drinks. Syrups, teas, tonic water, and beverages can be seen as early forms of nutraceuticals because they were considered to be beneficial for one's health.

The history and use of patent medicines is well worth reviewing as related to the development of nutraceuticals in the twenty-first century. Patent medicines from the nineteenth century were in the tradition of tonics and elixirs as restorative boosters. However, patent medicines differed in two ways. First, the medications were produced for a mass market, which did not require consumers to seek the advice of apothecaries or formularies on an individual basis. Second, the ingredients contained

---

GINGER GARLIC TEA WITH LIME AND HONEY

Ingredients: ginger root, garlic, water, lime or lemon juice, honey

This tea was first made for me by Jesus Mejia, who boiled sliced fresh ginger root and smashed garlic cloves in a pot of water. One can inhale the steam as the pot boils to enhance breathing—if one's nasal passage is stuffy—or to loosen phlegm. After boiling the ingredients for about 20 minutes, pour the tea into a cup and add fresh lime or lemon juice and honey to taste. This tea is healing and restorative for colds and flu.

---

mostly alcohol with derivatives of herbs and sometimes opium or cocaine. Rather than patenting the ingredients, which varied considerably, the bottle or pictorial advertisement was usually patented. The extravagant claims of patent medicine in the nineteenth century were not covered by oversight or regulation. At best, such medications were harmless, but frequently they were iatrogenic, even deadly, if consumed in large doses. The rampant promotion of patent medicine and inconsistent regulation from state to state led the federal government to begin overseeing food and drug production. In many ways, the rise of federal government organizations to set standards and oversee the production and consumption of patent medicine is parallel to the evolving story of dietary supplements and nutraceuticals in the twenty-first century.

Before there were food-based nutraceuticals, vitamins were taken as food supplements in tablet form. Vitamins were first taken for nutritional reasons, such as the prescription for sailors of citrus fruits to prevent scurvy. Vitamin deficiency and its associated diseases such as beriberi, pellagra, rickets, and scurvy were well known among nutritionists, yet it wasn't until seventeen vitamins were isolated during the first half of the twentieth century that scientists began to consider their health effects. Nobel laureate Linus Pauling advocated the consumption of vitamin C not only to prevent diseases like scurvy but also to reduce the risk of cancer and various other illnesses.

Since the second half of the twentieth century, vitamins as food supplements in tablet and powder form have become a form of self-medication. Supplements are currently an $11 billion industry in the United States. The 1994 Dietary Supplement Health and Education Act (DSHEA) urged the regulation of supplements not as additives but as food items.[1] The groundswell of popular support that led to the passage of this act reflects an ongoing concern about health care and the individual's access to medicinal foods or supplements. Noting that over 50 percent of Americans consumed some form of dietary supplement for nutritional reasons, the act outlined definitive terms for supplements and their claims, safety protections, and labeling guidelines. As of 2008, over a decade since the DSHEA, the supplement industry has more than doubled. Controversies concerning the efficacy of supplements and their safety reflect the terrain of contested knowledge of health and nutrition. Direct marketing to consumers has broadened the reach of both pharmaceuticals and supplements. Moreover, the use of vitamin supplements reflects individual ways of defining oneself, whether they are taken for muscle enhancement or metabolic rejuvenation.

Nutraceuticals follow the popular interest in naturally derived medicines from a very different angle. Nutraceuticals combine nutritional biochemistry with industrial food processing. Often the isolated compounds stem from natural products that have traditionally been consumed as food. Garlic, ginger, and ginseng, for instance, can be separately consumed in raw form, processed tablets, or with other food items. As nutraceuticals, these items may be found in combination with other food items such as beverages, candies, and desserts. Energy drinks, in particular, are a popular form of nutraceutical. New concoctions—such as Rock Star, Monster, and Red Bull—include a range of ingredients advertised as stimulants; they may include taurine, an amino acid found in animal bile, to aid digestion. Marine nutraceuticals have been developed extensively; fish oils, algae, chitin, glucosamine, and omega 3 fatty acids have been isolated in marine life and added to a range of foods.

For many consumers, nutraceuticals are just an extension of vitamins. Rather than requiring separate consumption of a vitamin or adding it to one's food, nutraceutical products are packaged as convenient and even delicious ways to enhance one's health. However, nutraceuticals differ from vitamins in that some products include items that may not occur as natural substances. Considerable efforts have been made to isolate compounds such as flavinoids (water-soluble plant pigments) that can be found in chocolate, wine, tea, strawberries, and raisins. Although flavinoid-rich foods have been associated with beneficial effects, the connection between flavinoid-enhanced foods and improved cardiovascular health has not been proven. The category of nutraceuticals draws on notions of natural foods, but the isolation of a compound to infuse a food through industrial processing is quite different from foods found in nature.

Nature's Medicine?

During the 1990s, there was great interest in harvesting the rich knowledge of traditional healers about medicinal plants.

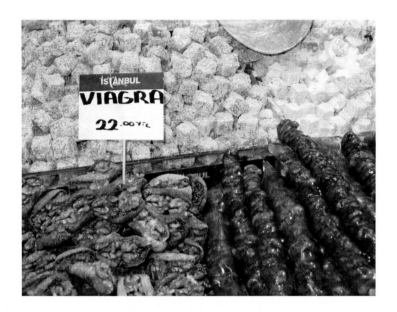

Figs inserted in walnuts next to carmelized sticks of walnuts advertised as food versions of Viagra, Egyptian spice market, Istanbul, 2006

Ethnobotanists, anthropologists, and other scientists comb tropical rain forests and coastal marine areas for medicines on the new front line of pharmaceuticals. Discoveries of the anti-cancer properties of the Pacific yew tree (*Taxus brevifolia*) led to the new cancer drug Taxol in 1991. The interest in medicines derived from nature has been driven by the lucrative promise of bioprospecting, the practice of developing drugs from bio-active ingredients in plants and living entities.

As the nutraceutical industry matures, questions of audience and access arise. The debate about who produces, buys, and consumes nutraceuticals will be critical to watch. With the development of such products in capital-intensive enterprises, the question of who consumes nutraceuticals will be crucial. Will nutraceuticals follow organic foods, which tend to be directed at the high end of markets, or will these products be made available to all consumers? As more nutraceutical products become available in local groceries, knowledge about nutrition on the part of consumers will also be key. Moreover, the industry faces very different questions of purity from the organic food movement and its regulation. Labeling foods as organic has been highly contested because organic growers and grassroots organizations hold that they have stricter guidelines on what is organic from the definition of organic by the federal government. Instead, the nutraceutical industry faces ongoing work to develop nutritional standards. Concerns for quality management, standardization, and substantiation of claims reflect concerns similar to those of dietary supplements.

The role of the FDA in shaping this industry is also an arena to watch. In 2002, the federal agency had several hearings on nutraceuticals to determine regulation for them. Many supporters held that such nontoxic foods with health benefits should be included in the category of supplements. In 2004, the FDA banned the Nutraceutical International Corporation from selling its products containing ephedra.[2] A series of deaths were linked to the herb, which was used in weight loss products and had amphetamine-like effects on the heart. After a year of litigation, U.S. District Judge Tena Campbell ruled in April 2005 that the FDA wrongly regulated this herb as a drug rather than as a food. Under DSHEA guidelines, a supplement company only needs to prove that a dietary supplement is harmful rather than prove it is safe as a drug. Industry watchers and consumers view this ruling as a reversal of the FDA ban. However, there remains a great need for public safety and mechanisms for assessing risk from dietary supplements.

Nutraceuticals are being closely watched elsewhere. In Japan, nutraceuticals sales are estimated to be as high as $30 billion per year (Yamaguchi, 2004). Nutritional products are in much demand despite the recession in Japan, where cultural notions of taking care of the mind and body with medicinal foods and dietary supplements remain quite popular. Tonics such as vitamin water and energy drinks with supplements continue to sell very well there. It is said that the category of functional foods first surfaced in Japan. Rather than using the term "functional foods," the label FOSHU (Foods for Specific Health Use; *tohuko* in Japanese) was introduced by the Japanese Ministry of Health, Labor, and Welfare in 1993. Used for 15 percent of functional foods on the market, this label indicates whether a food or drink has recognized health-benefiting ingredients. Acquiring the FOSHU label is voluntary. As long as a company does not advertise the product as beneficial for a particular disease, health-enhancing or health-supporting claims are allowed. The Japanese nutraceutical market is perhaps the largest in the world, with the average consumer spending twice as much as Americans and four times as much as Europeans on nutraceuticals. There are nearly 400 products with FOSHU labels, while many other healthy foods or medicinal products do not bear the label. In contrast to the FDA, Japanese regulation tends to emphasize labeling that is voluntary in a well-established yet expanding industry. In Asian markets, the overlapping relation between beverages and wellness drinks suggests an ambiguous location between medicine and health on one hand and taste and pleasure on the other. Nutraceuticals are viewed in Japan as not only healthy but also tasty.

The European Food Safety Authority (EFSA), based in Parma, Italy, monitors food and feed safety for the European Union using independent scientific studies that evaluate risk. In addition, the Health and Consumer Protection Directorate General, based in Brussels, monitors public health, food safety, and consumer affairs. The European focus on risk and concerns about safety offers more finely tuned approaches to understanding the broad spectrum of nutraceuticals. Yet, similar to the United States, there are advocacy groups such as the European Nutraceutical Association (ENA) based in Basel and devoted to examining the scientific basis of nutraceuticals since July 2005. Proclaimed as a partner to the American Nutraceutical Association, the ENA notes on its website that "the more knowledge is obtained about the health-promoting effect of foods, the more blurred this seemingly strict separating line becomes between these two product groups."[3]

These three different approaches to nutraceuticals reflect how the category is shaped relative to state regulation of pharmaceuticals, food, and dietary supplements. In what follows, I examine how recent legislation to harmonize or make uniform the standards for preparation, packaging, selling, and consumption of food supplements on a broader global scale will shape the nutraceutical industry.

Harmonization and Globalization

Harmonization is a process of aligning prior national or state regulations with recent international treaties and trade agreements. The process can also be viewed as an ongoing project of standardization for various practices and products on a global scale. To date, there have been regulatory bodies to oversee the harmonization of taxes, donor policies, environmental concerns, food safety, medical devices, magnetic fields, pharmaceuticals, and biotechnology among others. The European Union has had to develop many guidelines because of the diversity of its member nations. Asian countries have also participated in harmonization efforts, especially as members of regional and global trade agreements. Harmonization of standards for nutraceuticals has come in the form of the Codex Alimentarius, a United Nations commission charged to define and set guidelines on food standards and safety. Since 1963 the commission has set 243 food standards and 57 hygiene practice codes, in addition to setting pesticide residue levels and food additives.[4]

In July 2005, the Codex Alimentarius Commission met to discuss vitamin and mineral supplement guidelines for the World Trade Organization (WTO) and the General Agreement on Tariff and Trade (GATT) trade standards. The main issue was whether to follow recommended daily allowances (RDA) of supplement standards common in the United States or to adapt standards that were based on risk assessments more common in Europe. As the supplement industry in the United States is worth $11 billion, this would have huge effects, not only on domestic production but also on sales in the U.S.-based vitamin and food supplement industries.

Early reactions to Codex proposals from U.S. consumers and supplement companies raised concerns that the regulations would restrict the ability to purchase dietary supplements or the seemingly ubiquitous vitamin C tablets. Moreover, there was concern that the Codex would turn back the legislative actions of the DSHEA. In response, the FDA put out a list of facts clarifying its stance on the Codex and the benefits of compliance. In particular, the agency emphasizes that consumer access and domestic standards will not change overnight without the actions of Congress and the administration. Rather, the Codex is only a set of trade guidelines with a likely extended period of implementation. The main concern is less about domestic access than about the competitive ability of U.S.-made supplements in international commerce.

Harmonization of guidelines on food production and dietary supplements suggests that globalized standards are inevitable. However, even if nutraceuticals traverse commercial paths framed by trade agreements, the preference for local flavors and the search for new tastes suggest other ways in which regional and cultural practices shape how we consume medicine as food and in functional foods.

Nutraceuticals are nothing new in non-Western contexts. Rather than supposing a flow of nutraceuticals from the United States, many products have existed in Asian and Latin American markets for some time. These include energy drinks, present in Japanese and other Asian food markets for several decades. Any beverage vending machine in Japan, Taiwan, and South Korea likely stocks a range of drinks such as "Pocari Sweat" (an ion-supply drink to replace electrolytes lost in sweat), "Calpis" (a yogurt-based carbonated drink), iced coffee, iced green tea, milk tea, mineral water, and specially blended waters with royal jelly or vitamins. Many such drinks are viewed as prototypes for new products designed for the U.S. market. Supermarkets and convenience stores in the United States already offer a range of enhanced bottled water products such as vitamin water and "smart water."

In addition, a range of juices and fresh milks made from fruit seeds, ubiquitous in markets and street stalls throughout Asia and Latin America, offer new product possibilities. These include hemp milk, made from hemp seeds and similar to soy milk, which is a refreshing drink in tropical Asia. Plum soda and hawthorn juice, both sweet and tart, are also popular in Asia. Bubble tea, tea-based drinks with tapioca pearls or balls, and wheatgrass jelly from Taiwan have also become popular in the urban United States. Nutraceutical drinks that have been marketed and consumed in Asia or Latin America are being repackaged for Euro-American consumers. Acai, a tart Amazonian berry rich in antioxidants, has been packaged as a drink and as a flavoring for a range of foods in North America.

Thinking about nutraceuticals as part of a cultural system takes into account the ways in which this category has been shaped by various players: the industrial food system, the pharmaceutical industry, government regulators, international codes, and, not least, consumers. Concerns about health and the desire for well-being lead many consumers to seek out alternatives to processed foods that are less iatrogenic. Nutraceuticals address this concern by offering enhanced foods that seem more nutritious or supplements with specific health benefits for particular disorders. Rather than asking what is natural about nutraceuticals, it may be more fruitful to ask what the blurring of boundaries between medicine and food accomplishes. Can nutraceuticals enable better nutrition and, by extension, better health? Or will nutraceuticals enable better health only for those who can afford such products? In recent years, concerns for food safety has expanded as various industrial foods and globalized food economies open up new arenas for oversight. In what follows, I consider how boundaries between food and medicine further dissolve, while the categories at the same time overlap through genetic manipulation.

CHAPTER FOUR

Genetically Modified Food and Drugs

Genetically modified (GM) or genetically engineered (GE) foods have been present in industrial foodways for over a decade. Despite reluctance to accept GM foods worldwide, over two-thirds of processed foods in the United States include GM ingredients. Moreover, in the world's most populous countries, India and China, GM crops have been planted with the Malthusian perspective that this technology will prevent widespread hunger and dependency on foreign aid. Agricultural corporations claim that farmers in these regions find that GM crops decrease the need for pesticides as they increase crop yields. While knowledge about GM foods at the consumer level might be enhanced with new labeling practices, less well known is the increasing presence of GM and GE drugs. These have entered medicinal pathways following the slippery slope of the entry of genetically modified organisms (GMOs) in foodways. The previous chapter addressed how enhanced foods generated new blurrings of medicine as food. This chapter examines the continued transformation of food through genetic manipulation to enable new traits that supposedly are beneficial and even touted as medicinal. Most attention has previously been paid to GM food rather than GE drugs. As with nutraceuticals, new forms of medicinal production and consumption are also emerging from this process.

Here I examine cultural discourses concerning GM food and drugs, notions of purity, and meanings of risk, thereby enabling a broader framework for discussing GMOs in relation to notions of nation-making. Rather than asserting binary distinctions between Western and non-Western or developed and developing nations, the ubiquity of GMOs reflects how foodways and drugs are increasingly interconnected in a global context. Culture, politics, and knowledge influence the reception of GM products by consumers.

Responses toward GM foods have shifted in the past decade. The debate is usually framed in terms of being simply for or against these foods, but it is more productive to consider different views of GM foods in relation to the corporate, national, and consumer interests that shape their production and circulation. The corporate and industrial promotion of GM foods has strongly emphasized the progress of scientific technology and the benefits of bioscience in the advancement of life. Agribusiness interests portray GMOs as the solution to farmers' needs at the same time as they meet market demand for year-round produce or cheaper food. Responses toward GMOs from nation-states and governing agencies echo this discourse. There may be overlapping and even contradictory positions on GMOs within the same government.

Marion Nestle has documented the multiple agencies in the United States that are involved in food regulation (2003). Some government entities may embrace and promote the message of agribusiness interests—that GMOs meet markets' and farmers' needs to have a secure food supply all year round.

Other government agencies, however, focus on concerns of risk and the management of GM crops or products in foodways. The response during the 1990s was mostly to resist what the media has dubbed "frankenfoods." This response drew on notions of engineered foods as unnatural, impure, and dangerous. Initial consumer concerns were raised when milk produced from cows injected with recombinant bovine growth hormone (rBGH) was introduced into commercial milk production. The "flavr saver" tomato, an FDA-approved GE tomato designed to have a longer shelf life, had a short-lived market presence due to high costs and consumer disapproval. When traces of StarLink corn, intended as GM feed for animals, were found in fast foods intended for human consumption, the public began to be aware of the ubiquity of GMOs in the food chain. Many foods produced from GE seed or prepared with GE vegetable oil have made their way into the diet of people of all ages and backgrounds, in products ranging from infant formula to vitamin supplements. Genetically modified soy or corn, for instance, is added to a wide range of processed foods that use either vegetable oil or derivatives, including potato chips, hot dogs, chocolate, breakfast cereal, and even infant foods.

The discussion of GM foods has tended to focus on plant-based foods. Cloned animals, however, seem to raise the bar on public concerns with inclusion in human foodways and safety. Cloned livestock have been under specific evaluation since 2003 by the FDA. In January 2008, the agency released final cloning risk-assessment reports that deemed cloned cows, pigs, and goats safe for consumption and required no labeling.[1] The FDA consumer health update even pointed out that the majority of cloned livestock was primarily for the purpose of breeding stock rather than for consumption. Scientific experts note that young cloned calves may exhibit developmental problems such as unregulated temperatures; if they survive to later stages, however, these animals will eventually outgrow such problems and resemble their uncloned counterparts. Hence, veal from cloned cattle is not recommended. Although such products have yet to reach American markets, responses to GM foods and GM animals in human foodways depend greatly on social and political contexts that frame health risk from consumption of cloned meat to broader concerns of food shortage.

The discovery that many foods from the United States may have been produced with GE or GM seed, plant, or feed has led to a call for labeling of GE and GM products. Since 1999, international trade agreements have addressed the issue of harmonization of food labeling, and the FDA has supported voluntary rather than mandatory labeling practices for GM products. Some U.S. states have introduced legislation concerning GM labeling with mixed results. In 2005, Alaska became the first state to successfully require such labeling. A similar bill introduced in Oregon in 2002 failed to pass.

By contrast, European positions concerning GM food have been extensively documented in official European Union (EU) guidelines, as well as by nongovernmental organizations. In 2004, EU food regulators passed legislation on food labeling that will have significant changes beyond Europe, particularly for food producers and suppliers. The European emphasis on GM labeling seeks to manage GMOs by way of market principles and regulation. In 2005 Greenpeace published its own report, "No Market for GM in EU Markets," using so-called gene detectives to assess how well food distributors and retailers maintained an anti-GM policy; the detectives spot-check supermarket shelves. Guided by assessments of risk, labeling entails attention to several different arenas in which genetic manipulation takes place. All GM-derived products must be labeled even if no GM DNA is detectable in the final product. All plant, seed, feed, or other additives produced by a GMO must be noted. Such labeling laws help clarify the link between producers, distributors, and consumers. Moreover, the emphasis on tracking GMOs at multiple levels of the food chain, from plants to animals to humans, enables a multilevel view of GM in industrial foodways.

Living with GMOs as a presence in the foodways entails health risks and environmental hazards that include altering biodiversity. Considering risk as part of a cultural logic of daily life helps frame the difference between various countries' approaches to GM foods. In the Codex Alimentarius discussions of May 2005, it was clear that not all countries view GM foods the same way. The attempt to set up uniform guidelines in GM labeling failed, despite the fact that the majority (30 of 55) of participating countries, including France, the United Kingdom, India, and Brazil, favored standard labels. The United States and Argentina, the largest GM crop producers, did not agree to mandatory labeling standards. The risk model of labels presumes that GM foods are already in the foodways. It should be up to the *informed* consumer, this model argues, to decide whether to purchase or eat any food produced with genetic modification. Access to information and knowledge about GMOs mostly eludes ordinary consumers.

Risks to consumer health and the loss of biodiversity are not the only concerns raised when GM seeds are planted or when a GM policy is devised at the national level. Another cultural discourse of risk concerns a secure food source. The response to GM foods by developing nations is illuminating in this regard. In 1999, Thailand was among the first non-European nations to ban imports of GE seed. African nations such as Zambia, Malawi, Zimbabwe, and Angola also do not take GM seed or accept GM food when they are offered in aid programs, despite the famine and starvation in those countries. Emphasis on long-term concerns for biodiversity and avoiding further dependency on GM food or seed militate against the short-term aid of such items.

Feeding the Nation

Given the resistance against GM foods, what might be reasons for the embrace of GMOs in some nations? In China and India, the emphasis on a secure food source suggests a different consideration of food in terms of security and food for survival. Both countries face similar concerns: they must provide for largely rural populations of over a billion people in a context of global agribusiness that is increasingly influencing local agricultural practices. While both countries consider biotechnology as an element of nation building and food security, their responses to GMOs are somewhat different. The concerns for food security have transitioned from simply ensuring high food production to issues of food safety and food sovereignty in facilitating GM foods.

The Chinese state has much at stake in promoting biotechnology research and industry. Science and technology can rescue China from a Malthusian fate of too many people and not enough food. Widespread starvation in the aftermath of the Great Leap Forward, as well as famines in other times, remain deeply etched in personal and institutional memories. In such a context, biotechnology is a savior, not the problem that it is in Euro-American accounts. Biotechnology has been touted as the best solution for meeting the needs of the world's largest population, ranging from food shortages to health care concerns. Within the next three decades, the estimated Chinese population will increase to 1.6 billion, and food production must increase by at least 60 percent to match this growth. The aggressive promotion of this new science is deemed crucial, not only for material resources but also for the well-being of the nation.

An extension of this survivalist response is the concern about property in the race to the GMO patent finish line. Bureaucrats guided by the Communist government are determined not to become dependent on foreign aid relating to food. Such pressing concerns in this context outweigh the concerns for safety voiced in Europe and the Americas. Agricultural biotechnology is an extremely controversial area, and it has received extensive media coverage. In 1988, China became the first country to commercialize a bioengineered crop: a tobacco plant resistant to the tobacco mosaic virus. In 1999, the People's Republic of China invested $112 million in GMO research, ten times more than Brazil or India, though the figure is just 5 percent of what the United States invested. To make up for this, China planned to increase the investment by 400 percent by 2005. In 2006, investment actually reached $7.8 billion.

In the 11th five-year plan (2006–2010), the focus on Chinese biotechnology has turned to health care applications rather than to agricultural biotech. During 2000, China filed the largest number of patents on GMOs for crops including cotton, rice, wheat, soy, maize, peanuts, tobacco, and traditional medicinal herbs. The most significant GM crops are cotton, tobacco, and rice. In 2002, Chinese farmers planted 2.2 million hectares of GM cotton, an area twice the size of Belgium. Scientists have developed 141 transgenic plants, with 65 already approved for commercial use in China (compared with 50 in the U.S.). Also in 2002, the Beijing Genomics Institute published the rice genome sequence (*Oryza sativa* L. ssp. indica). Another way to measure volume is the amount invested by the government. Experts project that the majority of rice, wheat, corn, cotton, soy, and canola will be transgenic by 2010. In 2006, officials raised government funding of ag-biotech research to U.S. $500 million annually. This may be less than what some multinational firms invest, but yields come in the form of almost immediate harvests.

What does it mean to develop a GM crop? The most common GM traits bred in agricultural products include resistance to disease, bacteria, insects, and herbicides. Moreover, there is ongoing research in breeding sheep and goats with more meat; developing human vaccines in the milk of goats, rabbits, and cows; sequencing the pig genome; and successfully cloning goats and cows. At the same time, the Chinese government is also aware of external markets that do not want GMOs and has started to zone regions that are GMO-free for export to markets that seek this. Crop migration remains a problem. Moreover, farmers are accused of GM piracy in planting certain crops without waiting for permission.

It is instructive to pay attention to how GM cotton, rice, and soy in China feature different facets of state policy toward agricultural biotechnology. In 2001, over 4 million small-scale farmers planted Bt (*Bacillus thuringiensis*) cotton over 1.6 million hectares (up from 100,000 hectares in 1998), and these figures were expected to grow. By 2002, Chinese labs had developed 18 varieties of pest-resistant Bt cotton. GM rice is soon expected to follow GM cotton. China's genomic center in Beijing surprised the international science community with its quick sequencing of the rice genome two years ago.

Though soy originated in Asia and continues to be consumed in great quantities there, the contemporary reach of GM soy reveals multiple entanglements between global agribusiness empires, states, and consumers.

One story about soy is depicted in a 2004 advertisement run by Archer Midland Daniels, an American corporation that processes the majority of U.S. crops of corn, soy, and other agricultural products. The ad, which ran for several weeks in major American news journals such as *Newsweek* and *Time*, contains an image of a young Chinese boy with chopsticks facing a plate of tofu. The accompanying text states, "Somewhere west of Shenyang, a young Chinese boy is stopping for dinner. Which is why the soybean harvest west of Peoria is not stopping. And why a soybean processor west of St. Louis is not stopping. And why a ship's captain on the west coast is stopping, but just a while. Somewhere west of Shenyang a teenager is stopping for dinner. A dinner rich in protein. As one of world's largest soy processors, we like the idea there will be no stopping him now." The word "west" is repeated four times in this ad, and the concept of not stopping, or stopping only briefly, is also drummed home. The advertisement's message is that GM soy is feeding the new China.

Soy has a different trajectory than cotton or rice in China; rather than produce GM soy from its own seeds, China has been importing soybeans and soybean products from the United States—products derived from Roundup Ready soybean seedstock under a series of interim safety certificates, only recently issuing final ones. In a 2004 statement, American Soybean Association President Ron Heck of Perry, Iowa, clarifies:

> China's decision to issue final safety certificates for Roundup
> Ready soybeans is good news for U.S. farmers, as well as for

Chinese consumers who rely on imports of high quality soybeans to be processed into cooking oil and livestock feed. This action will help insure a steady market for U.S. soybeans, while helping stabilize meat, fish, egg, and cooking oil prices for Chinese consumers.[2]

Heck's statement was based on two years of field and food safety tests in China on the safety, healthfulness, and environment-friendliness of Roundup Ready soybeans. Soy is promoted as pure and healthy, drawing on scientific studies that link soy protein and isoflavones with reduced rates of chronic diseases such as heart disease, cancer, diabetes, and osteoporosis, in addition to alleviating menopausal conditions. Consumption of soy has risen dramatically in the past decade. Soy-based foods include not only tofu products and soy milk but also cooking oil, margarine, soy flour, and infant formula, among others. GE soy reaches well into industrial foodways at the same time that it is associated with health promotion.

Soy extends well beyond China and the United States. Part of the untold story of soy is that GM soy is poised to be the largest export crop in Latin America. Traditionally known for its cattle industry, Argentina has seen soy supplant beef as the largest export crop; observers now talk about soy republics instead of banana republics. GE soy edges out other plants that have been grown as food crops by local farmers in Latin America. The rise in GE soy is linked to the increased use of corn for ethanol production, and farmers in the United States have expanded corn cropland. This has led to the increased cultivation of soy crops throughout Latin American. Though it is also possible to develop soy as a biodiesel, the rise in consumption of soy in multiple forms ranging from soymilk or tofu to vegetarian hot dogs has also contributed to soy as a leading cash crop. The global consequences of this shift have led to increased fires and deforestation of the Amazonian rainforest for clearing more farmland for soy.[3]

Like China, India must meet the needs of a growing population of over a billion people. There are about two dozen GM crops in field trials in India, including rice, mustard, tomato, cabbage, cauliflower, and tobacco. Yet the response to GM foods has been different, in part due to India's experience with Monsanto. The agricultural company sold Indian farmers Bt cotton seeds, genetically modified to resist more pests and disease than conventional cotton. Farmers in southern India, particularly in Andhra Pradesh, saw their crops subsequently fail, causing them to lose their entire livelihoods in one season, in turn sparking a wave of suicides. Harvesting seed for the next crop, a traditional farming practice, has been challenged by Monsanto's proprietary stance toward GM seeds. Despite such concerns, the Genetic Engineering Approval Committee in the Ministry of Environment has approved of six new cotton hybrid plants. The volume of GM plants is not as high as in China. However the embrace of biotechnology in both of these countries will ensure increased reliance of GMOs, whether for domestic consumption or for export.

The decision to plant GMO crops is not an easy one. Developing countries do not passively accept the goal of multinational seed companies. Rather, the desire to be independent of import foods and to provide for large populations weighs heavily in making food security policy. Feeding a nation over time requires critical assessment of short-term goals of a secure food source and long-term goals of building nations from healthy citizens. In both China and India, the role of government oversight is crucial in determining which seeds are allowed for planting and which crops will be used for export or domestic consumption. The promise of GMOs suggests a rosy outcome of high-yield crops, fewer pesticides, and a bigger food supply. Farmers in both countries, however, face a different, less rosy, picture. The long-term effects of GMOs have yet to be documented. In response to anti–GM food sentiment elsewhere, China has developed organic crops to meet European and other Asian countries' preferences for GMO-free foods.

GE Drugs and Pharming

While GM foods have been a huge public concern for farmers and government agencies, GE drugs are only recently coming under public scrutiny. The applications of biotechnology have enabled new blurrings of food and medicine specifically via the production of genetically engineered drugs using conventional plants such as corn, soy, rice, and tobacco as substrates. These practices have been referred to as "pharming" (the production of pharmaceuticals via farming) or "biopharming," which is considered to be a cheaper form of recombinant drug production than conventional production processes. Plants and pharmaceuticals may be combined by way of technologies such as xenotransplantation, or the transplantation of genetic material from one species to another—most commonly, this is moving animal cells, tissues, or organs from animals into plants. Modified plants and animals can thus express traits that otherwise would not be seen. A sensational example included the production of human ears grown on the backs of laboratory mice. In pharmaceutical applications, genes for mostly proteins, antibodies, and other vaccines are inserted into plants or animals. The boom era of blockbuster drugs, or drugs that bring in over $1 billion a year, may be cut short by widespread concerns over some drugs' dangerous side effects, leaving lawsuits in its wake. Many Big Pharma drug companies, however, have been shifting to what is known as personalized medicine. The issue of tailor-made drugs by way of pharmacogenomics or biopharmaceuticals emphasizes drugs specific to an individual's genetic makeup. Concerns about the safety of generics or blockbuster drugs seem to have been sidestepped because such drugs are deemed to be genetically engineered for specific diseases and bodily reactions to drugs. As noted in chapter 3, functional foods or nutraceuticals are portrayed as enhancing nature, the essential properties of foods emphasized for more informed consumption. By contrast, genetically modified food and drugs are deemed unnatural and are made because of human intervention. GE drugs may be viewed with less concern than GM foods because food and drugs are held to be separate entities. GE drugs also differ from GM foods in that GE drugs do not seem far removed from other pharmaceuticals that are already produced in labs and factories. While tampering with food is highly charged, the greater distance of pharmaceuticals from food enables more interventions without cultural concerns about purity. Promoters of GE drugs learned an important lesson from the resistance to GM food. The cultural message of saving life or producing cancer-fighting drugs is very persistent.

Concerns about drug safety and efficacy continue to haunt both consumers and pharmaceutical companies. Even as GE drugs seem to promise a new era in medicine, there remain concerns about allergic reactions to human proteins introduced into plants. In the past two decades, over 100 GE drugs have been approved for market, several of which are blockbuster drugs. There are over 400 GE drugs in development by

Big Pharma. Despite extensive clinical trials, the safety of GE drugs is still inconclusive. For example, GE insulin has been linked with nearly 100 deaths from its use; nearly five times as many cases claim adverse reactions. The two largest pharmaceutical firms that control the market in insulin therapy phased out animal-based insulin products in favor of GE insulin, despite the high number of patients with adverse reactions. Animal-based biopharming is also subject to safety concerns. In late March 2008, the *New York Times* addressed contamination concerns in the global production of heparin, a commonly used blood thinner in surgery, by small pig-processing plants in China. The publication led to recalls of heparin by U.S., German, and Japanese companies.[4]

GE drugs intersect with GM foods in unique ways. There are now quite literal intersections between farms and Big Pharma in the making of GE drugs. GE pharming has been used in cultivating crops to produce edible vaccines. For instance, Australian biopharming has produced lettuce that has measles vaccines in it. Responses to animal tests have ranged from the positive outcomes (in which immune responses develop from consuming the transgenic plants) to more negative outcomes (in which allergic reactions emerge in response to proteins in a plant). In addition, there has been considerable concern about the use of corn in biopharming due to its easy assimilation into the human food chain. Instead, tobacco has been used in the new "pharm belt." Farms once engaged in less-lucrative crops such as tobacco production can now be cultivated for pharming new GE drugs. Environmental advocacy groups have raised concerns about pharm belt crossover where modified plants, mainly corn, may travel easily to pollinate food crops intended for human consumption without regulation.

GE drugs introduce an uncertain era in medicine, one in which personalized medicine is not about making existing medical systems or health care more accessible. Rather, medicine is within reach only for individuals who can afford it. Moreover, this kind of mixing of food and medicine neatly inverts the notion of food as medicine that we saw earlier. Eating food as the first line of healing, readily accessible to anyone with the knowledge or willingness, is embedded in the social and cultural traditions of medicine. What are the consequences of this shift toward medicines that become food based or produced via food crops? Those who believe in the purity of food and maintain strict boundaries between food and medicine may consider GM food and GE drugs to be perversions of nutrition and holistic medicine. GE drugs produced from biopharming are aligned with Big Pharma and agribusiness rather than local communities.

A consequence of the reaction against GM foods has been the increasing call for more organic choices and the absence of GMOs. The analogous call for drugs that are not GE has yet to be formulated. What is promoted as the sweet success of breakthroughs in biomedicine may instead become bitter medicine for consumers despite the promise of lower drug production costs.

As food and medicine become increasingly intertwined in production, market concerns in one arena will easily affect the other. When food crops such as corn or soy are converted to biopharming or the production of alternative fuel sources, unexpected market domino effects have led to rising food costs. Climate change has also exacerbated costs, leading to widespread food price increases across Asia, Africa, and Europe. Costs for basic staples such as rice, wheat, corn, cooking oil, and milk, among other foodstuffs, have risen in 2008, leading to food riots and protests across the globe. In response, the World Bank and the World Food Program are developing policies to help communities already facing deep poverty. Genetically modified food and drugs may continue to be promoted as necessary pathways to produce more for human consumption, despite ongoing concerns for safety.

Eating and Medicating

"Living to eat" is more suggestive of the possibilities of pleasure from consumption than more functional notions of "eating to live." Rather than maintain an anthropological distinction between eating for the good life or for survival, in this book I argue that eating with food as medicine in mind can dramatically shift the focus toward eating as part of a lifelong journey toward health. The quest for good health engages cultural knowledge, political formations, and blurred boundaries that redefine eating and medicating. Eating is not only about consuming food, it is also a social practice, often with political implications. The meanings of food and the associated politics of production and consumption are embedded in cultural frameworks that shape both everyday practices and important ritual moments. It is important to consider medicating as a cultural practice as well.

I use "medicating" instead of "healing" because I am referring to the specific act of consuming or treatment with a medicinal substance rather than the broader forms of healing practices that may range from holistic breathing exercises and physical therapy to more technology-based forms of treatment such as radiation and chemotherapy. Maintaining health begins with eating and understanding how food becomes categorized by cultural systems of knowledge. Rather than focus on defining food in moral categories of good to consume or bad to avoid, instead it is key to consider eating practices as part of broader health regimens.

Cultural Frameworks

Food is a conveyor of culture. It is often the first way in which people around the world experience healing at multiple levels. Health, wealth, and happiness are wishes often emblazoned in bold red characters at Chinese festivals and weddings. Celebratory feasts and wedding banquets across many cultures frequently include foods that are symbolic of fertility and prosperity. The linkage of health and wealth is not new. Spices in ancient Rome were copiously consumed, not only for medicinal purposes but also to show that one was wealthy enough to have access to such goods. Eating well in such cases reflected one's place in the world by way of foods that were equated with well-being. The cultural meanings of foods reflect moral and philosophical codes that shape social identities.

In traditional systems of healing, food was on the front line of medicine. Foods in the form of spices, healing broths, and elixirs were synonymous with medicine. This notion of medical or healing foods has persisted in many cultures. Following nutritional guidelines signals a different engagement with well-being. Eating to maintain health or deflect disease reflects an intimate process of forming identity or cultivating one's being by way of food and medicine. In such healing practices, health is viewed as a constant process rather than a steady state. Biomedicine gauges health in quantitative rates of blood pressure, heartbeats, cholesterol levels, and so on. An individual's measurements are compared with an average or a statistical standard to assess health in objective terms. Qualitative experiences of pain, suffering, and well-being are not as easily measured and hence are categorized as subjective and somehow less than real. As bodies vary greatly, those who have the same blood pressure reading—of 120 over 80—may have quite different body weights, metabolisms, and dietary needs. Nutritional guidelines offer standards and divide food into categories. As foods and medicines are being transformed by new technologies of production and processing, however, the notions of what makes good food or good medicine are being revised. Recent shifts in the production of industrialized food and medicine already greatly influence the choices we face.

In recent years, nutritional experts have urged both the general public and medical practitioners to promote nutritional literacy, particularly among children. Such calls for action are in response to growing nutritional illiteracy, especially in the awareness of diseases such as diabetes and cardiovascular disease that are preventable through nutrition. Nutritional knowledge has tended to focus awareness of numbers, as in calories, and also the ability to read and interpret labels. Such a reductionistic approach to food focused mainly on nutrients has been referred to as "nutritionism" (Pollan 2008).

In this book, I argue for a different kind of nutritional literacy, one in which consideration of food and medicine as cultural practices offers new possibilities for understanding how we consume on a social scale. Simple replication of ancient Greek diets or adoption of Chinese food therapy or any other system that has been popularized by the diet industry is inadequate; rather, diets or dietary regimens need further contextualization.

Consideration of the ethos of eating and medicating as part of daily life and regimen is critical. The quest for good health entails intimate knowledge of one's own health status, as well as situating eating and medicating practices within broader market formations of the industrial food complex, Big Pharma, and the diet industry.

Political Formations

Following Hippocrates, Galen frequently referred to all medicine as politics. In this book, I suggest that eating is similarly fraught with political implications. Greek physicians (*isonomia*) and Indian practitioners through Sanskrit translations referred to health as an ongoing search for equality (*samata*) in which physicians could establish justice through equilibrium between the humors (Zimmerman, 1987: 31). This notion of justice and equality, both at the microlevel of the body and in a social context, raises broader issues of social justice and access in a particularly compelling way. It offers insight into how health as a form of balance and equality is an important ideal and how this may inform practices of eating and medicating. The future of food, especially medicinal foods, will be greatly determined by issues of access, safety, and social justice. The maintenance of cultural knowledge in nutritional literacy and eating practices will also be critical.

Blurred Boundaries

The argument for blurred boundaries between food and medicine can have several consequences. In part I of this book,

I address the ways in which traditional medical systems link many forms of illness to environment and diet. The path to healing in this approach involves dietary interventions that can address the imbalance in one's body and daily regimen. Consuming foods to restore one's humors, cooking with spices, incorporating local or seasonal foods in one's diet, or eating with longevity in mind have been elements of medicinal foodways or dietary therapy. Dissolving boundaries between food and medicine in the contemporary moment, addressed in part II, suggests significant revisions in blurred lines between eating and medicating. The development of new foods introduced by the industrial food, pharmaceutical, and biotechnology industries may seem to address concerns about maintaining nutritional guidelines and food production. Indeed, broad concerns for food security or safety have shaped national agendas for food output. However, recent findings suggest that GMOs and nutraceuticals may have ecological and health impacts that are yet to be clearly defined and measured. As food crops are increasingly linked to energy resources, broader concerns for sustainability may also influence how we consume.

Food therapy has a long history, but in the present context of media bombardment, consumers are faced with conflicting expert information from all kinds of sources. Rather than mindlessly following the diet du jour, it is crucial to gain an innate sense and appreciation for how people eat and medicate in response to environmental and political conditions that continue to change. Rather than just focusing on *what* to eat, it is also crucial to consider *how* to eat, the latter greatly informed by cultural knowledge and practices. Attention to when one eats, where one eats, and with whom one eats can transform one's eating and ultimately medicating.

N O T E S

Introduction

1. For a recent report on nutrition in Finland, see http://www.ktl.fi/nutrition/. The Finnish National Public Health Institute documents a marked trend toward lower dietary fat consumption with more low-fat milk and dairy products produced and consumed.

Chapter 1

1. Though frequently used, the term TCM does not adequately address the dynamism of this system and how various theories and practices have transformed Chinese medicine. During the socialist era, Chinese medicine was directed to emphasize more uniform curricula and biomedical research practices rather than charismatic forms promoted by individual doctors. See Scheid (2002) for further discussion.

2. In Chinese medicine, the kidneys are considered the site where the essence of life is stored. The kidney itself is considered yin while its qi is yang. The balance of kidney qi influences reproduction, growth, and development. Any imbalance not only may lead to disruptions in these functions but also may manifest in a range of other pathologies. Gingko is believed to restore kidney yang energy.

3. For detailed U.S. Census age data information on baby boomers, see http://www.census.gov/population/www/socdemo/age.html.

Chapter 2

1. One such organization is the Salt Institute, which represents a consortium of salt producers and manufacturers. See http://www.saltinstitute.org/.

2. FDA Consumer, December 1997, http://www.fda.gov/fdac/features/1997/797_salt.html.

3. See www.nutrasweet.com/.

4. See www.stevia.net/.

5. See the white paper "Profitable Growth and Value Creation in the Soft Drink Industry: A View from Deloitte and SAP." Downloaded on July 20, 2006, from www.deloitte.com/dtt/article/0,1002,sid%253D52892%2526cid%253D91451,00.html.

6. See Harold Salzman, Roy Levy, and John Hilke, "Transformation and Continuity: The U.S. Carbonated Soft Drink Bottling Industry and Antitrust Policy Since 1980," Bureau of Economics Staff Report, Federal Trade Commission, November 1999. Downloaded on July 20, 2006, from www.ftc.gov/reports/softdrink/softdrink.pdf.

7. In 1981, the FDA noted that aspartame was safe to use in foods and has not determined any safety problems, despite allegations of adverse reactions. Updated May 2004. Downloaded on July 20, 2006, from http://www.cfsan.fda.gov/~dms/qa-adf9.html.

8. Marketdata Report no. FS22 "U.S. Weight Loss & Diet Control Market (9th Edition)" April 2007. See *http://www.mkt-data-ent.com /studies.html* and *http://www.marketdataenterprises.com/FullIndustryStudies. htm#WEIGHT* downloaded on July 25, 2008.

Chapter 3

1. Dietary Supplement Health and Education Act (DSHEA), available at http://www.fda.gov/opacom/laws/dshea.html.

2. Available at http://www.fda.gov/oc/initiatives/ephedra/february2004/.

3. See http://www.enaonline.org/index.php?lang=en&path&e quals;ueber_ena, downloaded March 30, 2008.

4. Codex Alimentarius, available at http://www.codexalimentarius. net/web/index_en.jsp.

Chapter 4

1. See http://www.fda.gov/bbs/transcripts/2008/cloning_transcript011508 .pdf, downloaded March 30, 2008.

2. Beam Beat. The American Soybean Association, "ASA Welcome Final Safety Certification of Roundup Ready Event in China." April 2004, p. 1. *http://www.soygrowers.com/publications/beanbeat/2004/Bean%20Beat% 20April%202004-final.pdf*, downloaded on August 12, 2008.

3. *Science* 318, no. 5857 (December 14, 2007): 1722.

4. David Barboza and Walt Boganich, "Twists in Chain of Supplies for Blood Drug," *New York Times*, February 28, 2008.

BIBLIOGRAPHY

Allen, Brigid, ed. 1994. *Food: An Oxford Anthology*. Oxford: Oxford University Press.

Alter, Joseph S., ed. 2005. *Asian Medicine and Globalization*. Philadelphia: University of Pennsylvania Press.

American Soybean Association. 2004. "ASA Welcomes Final Safety Certification of Roundup Ready Event in China." February 23. At http://www.soygrowers.com/newsroom/releases/2004%20 releases/r022304.htm.

Ames, Bruce N., and Lois Swirsky Gold. 1998. "The Causes and Prevention of Cancer: The Role of Environment." *Biotherapy* 11, no. 2/3: 205–20.

Anderson, E.N. 1988. *The Food of China*. New Haven, Conn.: Yale University Press.

Atkins, Peter, and Ian Bowler. 2001. *Food in Society: Economy, Culture, Geography*. London: Arnold.

Aubaile-Sallenave, Francoise. 2000. "*Al-Kishk.*" In Sami Zubaida and Richard Tapper, eds., *A Taste of Thyme: Culinary Cultures of the Middle East*. London: Tauris Parke.

Azmi, Altaf Ahmad. 1995. *Basic Concepts of Unani Medicine: A Critical Study*. New Delhi: Department of History of Medicine, Faculty of Medicine, Jamia Hamdard.

Barboza, David, and Walt Bogdanich. 2008. "Twists in Chain of Supply of Blood Drug." *New York Times*, February 28.

Bianque. 1986. *Nan-ching: The Classic of Difficult Issues, with Commentary by Chinese and Japanese Authors from the Third through the Twentieth Century*. Translated by Paul U. Unschuld. Berkeley: University of California Press.

Bourdieu, Pierre. 1984. *Distinction: A Social Critique of the Judgement of Taste*. Translated by Richard Nice. Cambridge, Mass.: Harvard University Press.

Bowker, Geoffrey C., and Susan Leigh Starr. 1999. *Sorting Things Out: Classification and Its Consequences*. Cambridge, Mass.: MIT Press.

Bright, Kristy. 1998. "The Traveling Tonic: Tradition, Commodity, and the Body in Unani (Greco-Arab) Medicine in India." Ph.D. diss., University of California at Santa Cruz.

Brillat-Savarin, Jean Anthelme. 1999 [1949]. *The Physiology of Taste, or, Meditations on Transcendental Gastronomy*. Translated by M. F. K. Fisher. Washington, D.C.: Counterpoint Press.

Buell, Paul D., Eugene N. Anderson, and Charles Perry. 2000. *A Soup for the Qan: Chinese Dietary Medicine of the Mongol Era, as Seen in Hu Szu-hui's Yin-shan cheng-yao. Introduction, Translation, Commentary, and Chinese Text*. London: Kegan Paul.

Buttress, Judy, and Mike Saltmarsh, eds. 2000. *Functional Foods II: Claims and Evidence*. Cambridge: Royal Society of Chemistry.

Caplan, Pat, ed. *Food, Health, and Identity*. 1997. New York: Routledge.

Cheng, Yuan. 2001. *Yao Wang Sun Simiao Chuan Qi* (Medical King Sun Simiao Legacy). Beijing: People Literature Press.

Codex Alimentarius Commission. 2005. *Report of the Thirty Third Session of the Codex Committee on Food Labelling*. May 9–13. At http://www.codexalimentarius.net/web/archives.jsp?year=05.

Cooper, Ann, with Lisa M. Holmes. 2000. *Bitter Harvest: A Chef's Perspective on the Hidden Dangers in the Foods We Eat and What You Can Do About It*. New York: Routledge.

Counihan, Carole, and Penny Van Esterik, eds. 1997. *Food and Culture: A Reader*. New York: Routledge.

Dean, Kenneth. 1993. *Taoist Ritual and Popular Cults of Southeast Asia*. Princeton, N.J.: Princeton University Press.

Dominy, Nathaniel. 2004. "Fruits, Fingers, and Fermentation: The Sensory Cues Available to Foraging Primates." *Integrative and Comparative Biology* 44: 295–303.

Douglas, Mary. 1984 [1966]. *Purity and Danger: An Analysis of Concepts of Pollution and Taboo.* London: Ark.

Douglas, Mary. 1986. *How Institutions Think.* Syracuse, N.Y.: Syracuse University Press.

Dupuis, E. Melanie. 2002. *Nature's Perfect Food: How Milk Became America's Drink.* New York: New York University Press.

Dupuis, E. Melanie. 2007. "Angels and Vegetables: A Brief History of Food Advice in America." *Gastronomica: The Journal of Food and Culture* 7, no. 3 (Summer): 000–000.

Elias, Norbert. 1982. *The Civilizing Process: The History of Manners.* Translated by Edmund Jephcott. New York: Pantheon.

Ernst, Waltraud, ed. 2002. *Plural Medicine, Tradition, and Modernity, 1800–2000.* New York: Routledge.

Etkin, Nina L., ed. 1994. *Eating on the Wild Side: The Pharmacologic, Ecologic, and Social Implications of Using Noncultigens.* Tucson: University of Arizona Press.

Etkin, Nina L. 2006. *Edible Medicines: An Ethnopharmacology of Food.* Tucson: University of Arizona Press.

Farquhar, Judith. 2002. *Appetites: Food and Sex in Postsocialist China.* Durham, N.C.: Duke University Press.

Fields, Gregory P. 2001. *Religious Therapeutics: Body and Health in Yoga, Āyurveda, and Tantra.* Albany: State University of New York Press.

Flandrin, Jean-Louis, Massimo Montanari, and Albert Sonnenfeld, eds. 1999. *Food: A Culinary History from Antiquity to the Present.* Translated by Clarissa Botsford, Arthur Goldhammer, Charles Lambert, Frances M. López-Morillas, and Sylvia Stevens. New York: Columbia University Press.

Foust, Clifford M. 1992. *Rhubarb: The Wondrous Drug.* Princeton, N.J.: Princeton University Press.

Galen. 2000. *Galen: On Food and Diet.* Translated by Mark Grant. London: Routledge.

Gladney, Dru C. 2003. "Resisting Food." Keynote address presented at the conference "Eat, Drink, Halal, Haram: Food, Islam, and

Society in Asia," Asia Research Institute and Department of Sociology, National University of Singapore, December 3–5.

Gladney, Dru C. 2004. *Dislocating China: Reflections on Muslims, Minorities, and Other Subaltern Subjects.* Chicago: University of Chicago Press.

Glosser, Susan L. 2003. *Chinese Visions of Family and State, 1915–1953.* Berkeley: University of California Press.Goodman, Alan H., Darna L. Dufour, and Gretel H. Pelto, eds. 2000. *Nutritional Anthropology: Biocultural Perspectives on Food and Nutrition.* Mountain View, Calif.: Mayfield.

Harris, Marvin. 1985. *Good to Eat: Riddles of Food and Culture.* New York: Simon and Schuster.

Hippocrates. 2005. *Hippocrates on Ancient Medicine.* Translated by Mark J. Schiefsky. Leiden: Brill.

Ho, Chi-tang, Jen-kun Lin, and Qun Yi Zheng, eds. 2003. *Oriental Foods and Herbs: Chemistry and Health Effects.* Washington, D.C.: American Chemical Society.

Hoffman, Jay M. 1997 [1968]. *Hunza: Secrets of the World's Healthiest and Oldest Living People.* El Monte, Calif.: New Win.

Holt, Mack P., ed. 2006. *Alcohol: A Social and Cultural History.* Oxford: Berg.

Ibn Qayyim Al-Jawziyah. 1994. *Natural Healing with the Medicine of the Prophet: From the Book of the Provisions of the Hereafter by Imam Ibn Qayyim Al-Jawziyya.* Translated by Muhammad Al-Akili. Philadelphia: Pearl.

Ibn Sinā [Avicenna]. 1996. *al-Qanun al-Tibb* (Canon of Medicine). Frankfurt: Institute for the History of Arabic-Islamic Science, Johann Wolfgang Goethe University.

Ibn Sinā [Avicenna]. 1970 [1930]. *A Treatise on the Canon of Medicine of Avicenna, Incorporating a Translation of the First Book.* Translated by O. Cameron Gruner. New York: Kelley.

Jank, Joseph K. 1915. *Spices: Their Botanical Origin, Their Chemical Composition, Their Commercial Use.* St. Louis: [Curran].

Johnston, Francis E., ed. 1987. *Nutritional Anthropology.* New York: Liss.

Kittler, Pamela Goyan, and Kathryn P. Sucher. 2001. *Food and Culture.* 3rd ed. Belmont, Calif.: Wadsworth.

Kotz, K., and M. Story. 1994. "Food Advertisements During Children's Saturday Morning Television Programming: Are They Consistent with Dietary Recommendations?" *Journal of the American Dietetic Association* 94: 1296–1300.

Kuriyama, Shigehisa. 1999. *The Expressiveness of the Body and the Divergence of Greek and Chinese Medicine.* New York: Zone Books.

Kurlansky, Mark, ed. 2002a. *Choice Cuts: A Savory Selection of Food Writing from Around the World and Throughout History.* New York: Ballantine.

Kurlansky, Mark. 2002b. *Salt: A World History.* New York: Walker.

Lachance, P. A., and R. G. Saba. 2002. "Quality Management of Nutraceuticals, Intelligent Product Delivery Systems and Safety through Traceability." In C.-T. Ho and Z. Zheng, eds., *Quality Management of Nutraceuticals.* Washington, D.C.: American Chemical Society, 2–9.

Lad, Vasant Dattatray. 2003. *The Philosophical and Fundamental Principles of Ayurveda.* Albuquerque, N.M.: Ayurvedic Press.

Laszlo, Pierre. 2001. *Salt: Grain of Life.* Translated by Mary Beth Mader. New York: Columbia University Press.

Li, Changfu, and Li Huiyan. 2003. *Sun Simiao Yang Sheng Quan Shu* (Sun Simiao Longevity Boxing). Beijing: Social Science Document Press.

Lin, Biing-hwan, and Kathryn Ralston. 2003. *Competitive Foods: Soft Drinks vs. Milk.* Food and Nutrition Research Report No. FANRR 34-7. Washington, D.C.: Department of Agriculture, Economic Research Service.

Lindenbaum, Shirley. 1979. *Kuru Sorcery: Disease and Danger in the New Guinea Highlands.* Palo Alto, Calif.: Mayfield.

Liu Jilin and George C. Peck, eds. 1995. *Chinese Dietary Therapy.* New York: Churchill Livingstone.

Lloyd, G. E. R. 1996. *Adversaries and Authorities: Investigations into Ancient Greek and Chinese Science.* Cambridge: Cambridge University Press.

Lloyd, G. E. R. 2003. *In the Grip of Disease: Studies in the Greek Imagination.* Oxford: Oxford University Press.

Lloyd, Geoffrey, and Nathan Sivin. 2002. *The Way and the Word:*

Science and Medicine in Early China and Greece. New Haven, Conn.: Yale University Press.

Lorde, Audre. 1982. *Zami: A New Spelling of My Name.* Watertown, Mass.: Persephone.

Mead, Margaret. 1997. "The Changing Significance of Food." In Carole Counihan and Penny Van Esterik, eds., *Food and Culture: A Reader.* New York: Routledge

McCarrin, Robert. 1922. "Faulty Food in Gastro-intestine Disorders." *Journal of the American Medical Association,* January 7.

Menzel, Peter, and Faith D'Aluisio. 2005. *Hungry Planet: What the World Eats.* Berkeley, Calif.: Ten Speed Press.

Miller, Daniel, ed. 1995. *Acknowledging Consumption: A Review of New Studies.* London: Routledge.

Miller, Daniel, ed. 1998. *Material Cultures: Why Some Things Matter.* Chicago: University of Chicago Press.

Miller, J. Innes. 1969. *The Spice Trade of the Roman Empire, 29 B.C. to A.D. 641.* Oxford: Clarendon.

Mintz, Sidney. 1986. *Sweetness and Power: The Place of Sugar in Modern History.* New York: Penguin.

Mintz, Sidney. 1996. *Tasting Food, Tasting Freedom: Excursions into Eating, Culture, and the Past.* Boston: Beacon.

Nair, C. K. N., and N. Mohanan. 1998. *Medicinal Plants of India: With Special Reference to yurveda.* Delhi: Nag.

Nestle, Marion. 2002. *Food Politics: How the Food Industry Influences Nutrition and Health.* Berkeley: University of California Press.

Nestle, Marion. 2003. *Safe Food: Bacteria, Biotechnology, and Bioterrorism.* Berkeley: Berkeley: University of California Press.

Ninivaggi, Frank John. 2001. *An Elementary Textbook of yurveda: Medicine with a Six Thousand Year Old Tradition.* Madison, Conn.: Psychosocial Press.

Oliver, J. Eric. 2006. *Fat Politics: The Real Story Behind America's Obesity Epidemic.* Oxford: Oxford University Press.

Petrini, Carlo. 2001. *Slow Food: The Case for Taste.* Translated by William McCuaig. New York: Columbia University Press.

Pollan, Michael. 2008. *In Defense of Food: An Eater's Manifesto.* New York: Penguin.

Rosenthal, Franz. 1990. *Science and Medicine in Islam: A Collection of Essays*. Brookfield, Vt.: Gower.

Sabur Ibn Sahl. 2003. *The Small Dispensatory: Translated from the Arabic, Together with a Study and Glossary*. Translated by Oliver Kahl. Leiden: Brill.

Sachs, Robert. 2002. *Tibetan yurveda: Health Secrets from the Roof of the World*. Rochester, Vt.: Healing Arts Press.

Sadler, Michèle J., and Michael Saltmarsh, eds. 1988. *Functional Foods: The Consumer, the Products, and the Evidence*. Cambridge: Royal Society of Chemistry.

Scheid, Volker. 2002. *Chinese Medicine in Contemporary China: Plurality and Synthesis*. Durham, N.C.: Duke University Press.

Schivelbusch, Wolfgang. 1992. *Tastes of Paradise: A Social History of Spices, Stimulants, and Intoxicants*. Translated by David Jacobson. New York: Pantheon.

Shahidi, Fereidoon, and Deepthi K. Weerasinghe, eds. 2004. *Nutraceutical Beverages: Chemistry, Nutrition, and Health Effects*. Washington, D.C.: American Chemical Society.

Shahidi, Fereidoon, Chi-tang Ho, Shaw Watanabe, and Toshihiko Osawa, eds. 2003. *Food Factors in Health Promotion and Disease Prevention*. Washington, D.C.: American Chemical Society, .

Sivin, Nathan. 1995a. *Medicine, Philosophy, and Religion in Ancient China: Researches and Reflections*. Brookfield, Vt.: Variorum.

Sivin, Nathan. 1995b. *Science in Ancient China: Researches and Reflections*. Brookfield, Vt.: Variorum.

Tannahill, Reay. 1989. *Food in History*. New York: Crown.

Tao Hong-jing. 1998. *The Divine Farmer's Materia Medica: A Translation of the Shen Nong Ben Cao Jing*. Translated by Yang Shou-zhong; edited by Bob Flaws. Boulder, Colo.: Blue Poppy Press.

Tufts, James W. 1895. *Book of Directions for Setting and Operating Soda-Water Apparatus: With Syrup Formulas and Miscellaneous Information*. Boston: Author.

Unschuld, Paul U. 1985. *Medicine in China: A History of Ideas*. Berkeley: University of California Press.

Unschuld, Paul U. 1986. *Medicine in China: A History of Pharmaceutics*. Berkeley: University of California Press.

Unschuld, Paul U. 2003. *Huang Di nei jing su wen: Nature, Knowledge, Imagery in an Ancient Chinese Medical Text*. Berkeley: University of California Press.

Watson, James L., ed. 2006. *Golden Arches East: McDonald's in East Asia*. 2nd ed. Stanford, Calif.: Stanford University Press.

Watson, James L., and Melissa L. Caldwell, eds. 2005. *The Cultural Politics of Food and Eating: A Reader*. Malden, Mass.: Blackwell.

Willcox, Bradley J., D. Craig Willcox, and Matsuo Suzuki. 2004. *The Okinawa Diet Plan: Get Leaner, Live Longer, and Never Feel Hungry*. New York: Clarkson Potter.

Yamaguchi, Paul. 2004. "Japan's Nutraceuticals Today: End of Year Japanese Nutraceutical Industry Thoughts and Looking Beyond. 2004-12-17." Available at http://www.npicenter.com/anm/templates/newsATemp.aspx?articleid = 11309&zoneid = 45.

Yang, Shou-Zhong. 1998. *Shen Nong Ben Cao Jing* (The Divine Farmer's Materia Medica Classic). Taos, NM: Redwing Books.

Yu J., Hu S., Wang J., Wong G. K., Li S., Liu B., et al. 2002. "A Draft Sequence of the Rice Genome (*Oryza sativa* L. ssp. Indica)." *Science* 296(5565): 79–92.

Zhang, Qifa. 1999. "China: Agricultural Biotechnology Opportunities to Meet the Challenges of Food Production." In G. J. Persley and M. M. Lantin, eds., *Agricultural Biotechnology and the Poor: Proceedings of an International Conference*, Washington, D.C., 21–22 October. At www.cgiar.org/biotech/repo100/Zhang.pdf.

Zimmerman, Francis. 1987. *The Jungle and the Aroma of Meats: An Ecological Theme in Hindu Medicine*. Berkeley: University of California Press.

Zubaida, Sami, and Richard Tapper, eds. 2000. *A Taste of Thyme: Culinary Cultures of the Middle East*. London: Tauris Parke.

INDEX